sharing life

inspiring stories of transplant patients and
their lifesaving heroes

Copyright © WMDA 2015

Published by WMDA
Email: mail@wmda.info
Website: www.wmda.info

Produced by Armour Publishing
Email: enquiries@armourpublishing.com
Website: www.armourpublishing.com

Cover photo by Monique Jöris

All rights reserved

No part of this publication may be reproduced, stored in a retrieval system or transmitted, in any form or by any means, electronic, mechanical, photocopying, recording or otherwise, without the prior permission of the copyright owner.

Printed in Singapore

ISBN: 978-981-4668-42-2

Contents

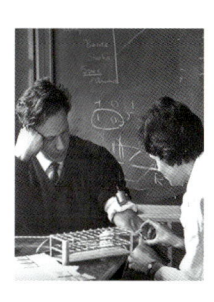

Introduction — vi

Section 1: Early pioneers

In the right place, at the right time — 3
Proud — 15
Miracle match — 23
Blazing trails in cord blood transplantation — 29
Planting a seed — 33
Recruiting unique genetics — 35

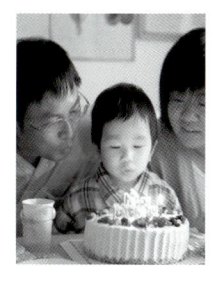

Section 2: Precious beyond words

"No big deal" — 41
Courage and commitment — 45
Let's proceed — 49
To my saviours — 51
Always moving forward — 53
Birthday gifts for Boris — 57
Fighting a battle on two fronts — 61
Search for meaning — 65
New perspectives — 69
Running mates — 73
Miracles of life — 75
Traces of you: A tale of love found, lost, then found again — 79
An open letter — 84

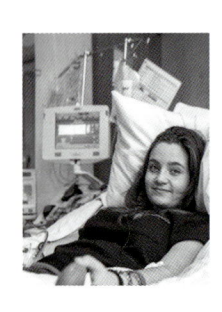

Section 3: The gift of giving

One match, two winners	89
A unique gift	95
A very special birthday gift	97
Finding Julie	101
Virtue, not duty	103
A family affair	107
The journey	111
Passion and perseverance	115
The kindness of strangers	119
A chance meeting	123
From China with love	125
A birthday surprise	129
World's youngest donor	133
Happiness and gratitude	137
Third time lucky	141
No longer strangers	143

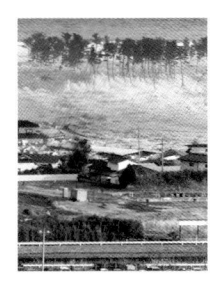

Section 4: Making the journey

From one mother to another	149
Last flight out of Atlanta	153
Dealing with super typhoon Haitang	157
Into the eye of the storm	161
Planes, trains and automobiles	167
From Washington DC to Wellington NZ in 72 hours	171
Great East Japan earthquake	175
Keep calm and courier on	179
Stepping up	183
Keeping our heads above the water	187
Collaboration across borders	189

Summary	193
Acknowledgements	195
Contributing registries	197
Glossary	207

Introduction

This is a book of cooperation, courage, resilience and hope. It is a collection of true stories that have happened, and are happening, all over the world.

Each contribution is a personal account of how someone who cares has reached across boundaries of nationality, ethnicity and geography to make a real difference to the life of another person. Each chapter in this book tells the story of how life is literally being shared every day through the gift of blood stem cells from one individual to another. They are narratives of how stem cell donors, doctors and registries have worked together to enable a global exchange and cooperation that has helped hundreds of thousands of patients worldwide.

Since the first bone marrow transplant in the 1950s, a staggering number of over a million transplants have been carried out. Bone marrow transplants are essentially transplants of blood-forming stem cells, and these patients received their transplants for the treatment of a wide variety of blood cancers and other diseases of the blood and bone marrow. While there have been many advances in the treatment of cancer and blood diseases, for many of these patients, blood stem cell transplants using healthy cells from a donor may be their only chance of a cure. Haematopoietic stem cell transplants (HSCTs) are transplants using bone marrow, blood-derived stem cells or cord blood stem cells from a donor that are sufficiently matched with the patient. When there is no suitable donor within a family, an unrelated donor, who could be from a completely different part of the world, will have to be found. That is when the registries associated with the WMDA step in and find that best match. They then facilitate notification of the donor, harvesting of the cells and their transportation, often across the world, to the patient. In fact, nearly 20,000 transplants are facilitated by these registries every year.

When we first embarked on the journey of writing this book, we knew it would be something special. We had heard of some extraordinary efforts being made in facilitating transplants, and we had also heard each other speak about our own deeply moving experiences with patients and donors. We knew we had an important story to tell and an important message for the world. So, in 2013, we sent out a call for stories from patients, donors, doctors, registry personnel and anyone who had been a part of facilitating a HSCT from an unrelated donor or cord blood unit. When the stories came in, we were overwhelmed. Each was a deeply personal account of how an individual had been moved in a very special way by his/her experiences. Each story reinforced our faith in humanity and the importance of the work we do every day.

In this book, you will read about a nurse who spent her 21st birthday in a very unique way; about a patient who was determined not to let his transplant get in the way of running a marathon; about a mother who fell on her knees when she saw the person who was carrying the cells that would save her child; and about the many heroes who braved natural disasters and emergencies to bring precious life-saving stem cells to someone in need.

In early 2015, the 25th million stem cell donor was recruited. Imagine that, 25 million people are willing to give their blood-forming stem cells to save another human being. It is our hope that this book will open your eyes to the fascinating world of stem cell transplants and renew your belief in the power of the human spirit.

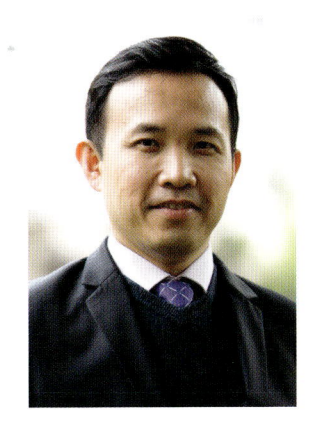

William Hwang
President (2013–2014), WMDA
Senior Consultant and Head,
Haematology, Singapore General Hospital
Director, SingHealth Transplant
Associate Professor,
Duke-NUS Graduate Medical School
Medical Director, Singapore Cord Blood Bank

Bardie
Starkie
Spec
d'America

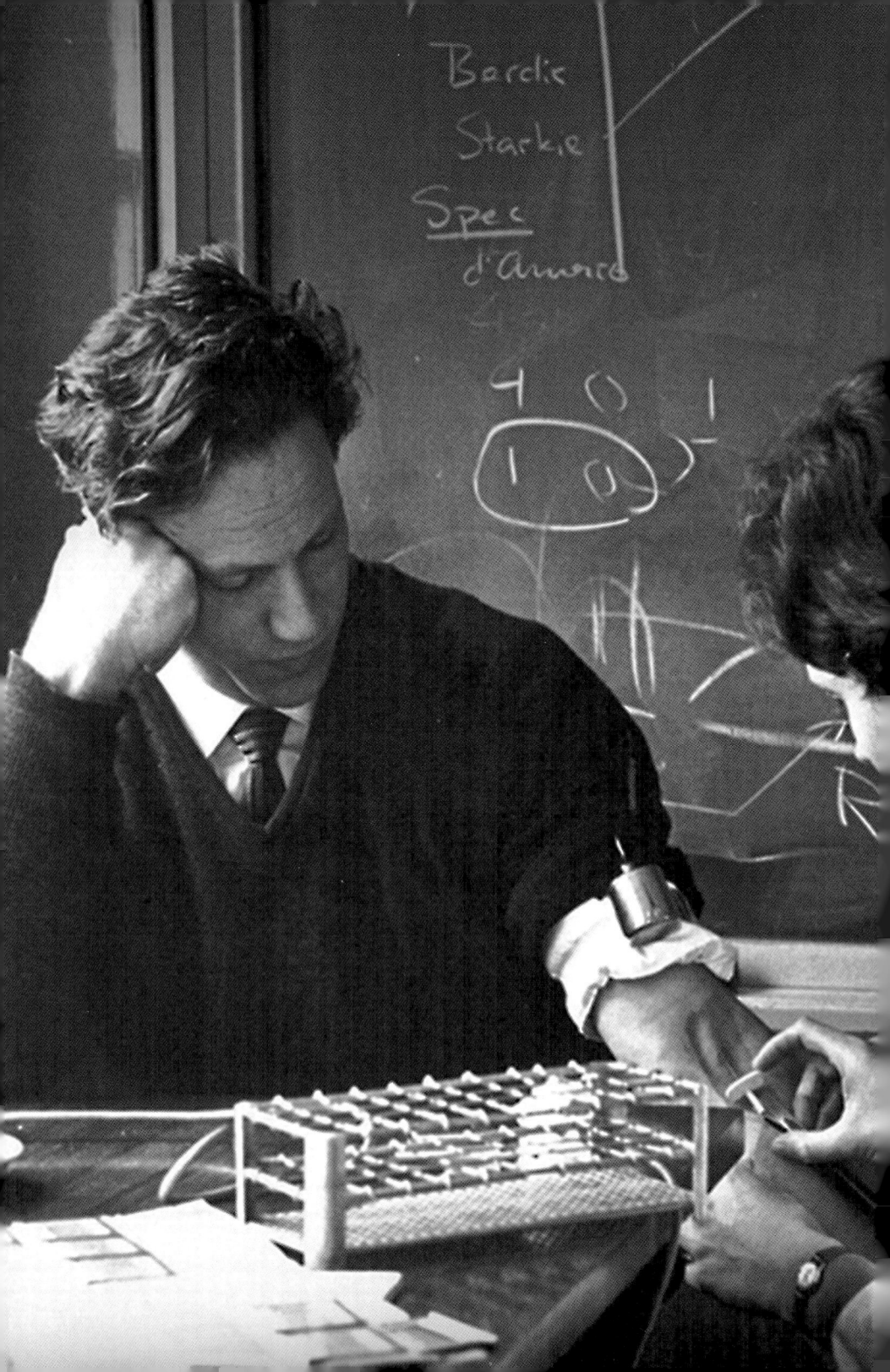

Section 1
Early pioneers

◀ Founding father of the WMDA Jon van Rood (left) and his life-long assistant Aad van Leeuwen (see Page 3 "In the right place, at the right time")

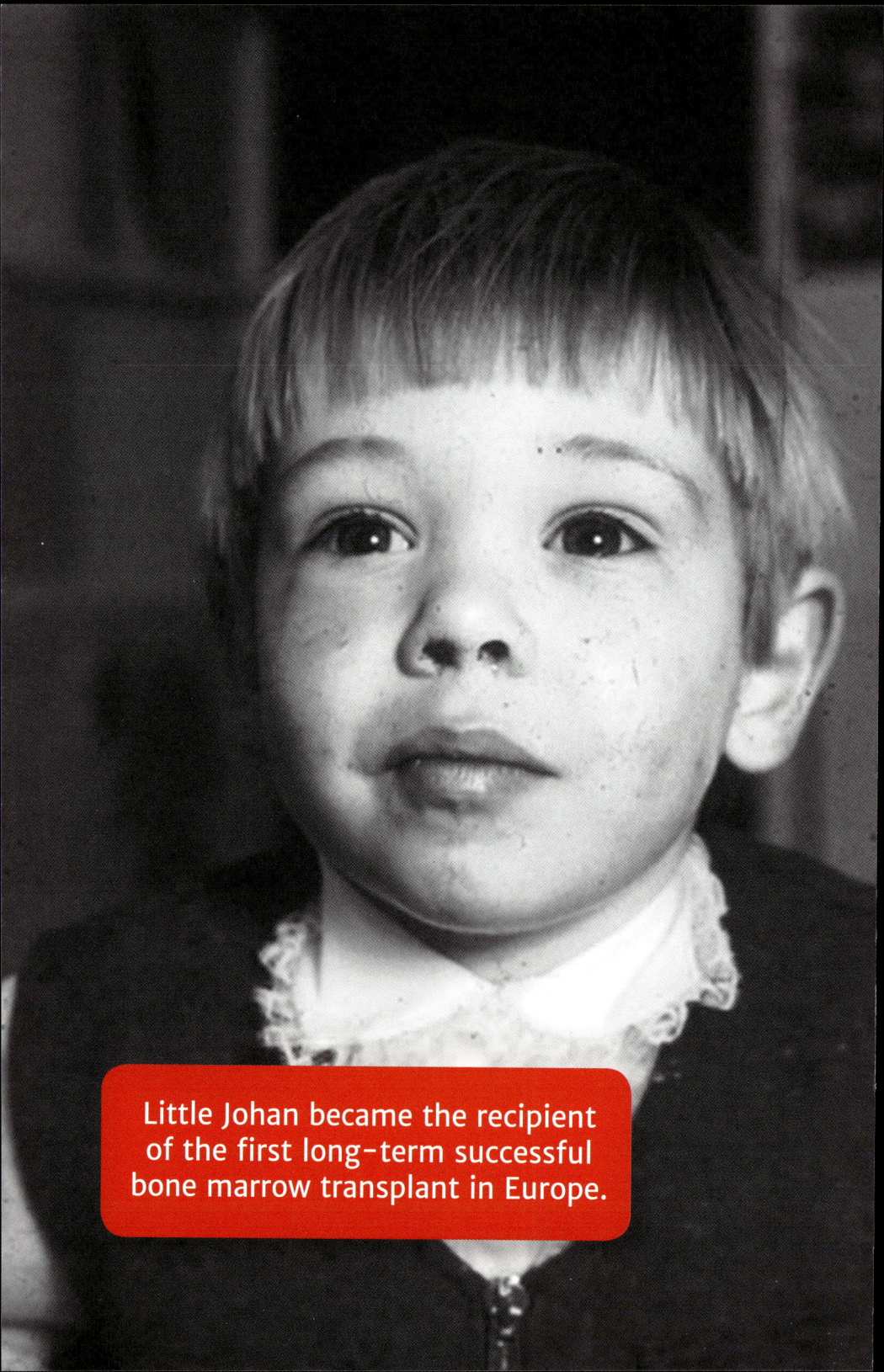

Little Johan became the recipient of the first long-term successful bone marrow transplant in Europe.

In the right place, at the right time

Prof Dr Jon van Rood, Co-Founder and President Emeritus of the WMDA

> In 2014, there were 110 unrelated stem cell donor registries and cord blood banks active in 65 countries around the world. Together they list more than 25 million donors and around 750,000 cord blood units available for patients in need. Worldwide, over one million transplants have been facilitated since this treatment was developed. International exchange has been, continues to be and will remain key to the success of blood stem cell transplantation.
>
> It all began more than 60 years ago with a handful of pioneers who had the vision, drive and passion to pursue a controversial treatment and—what was even more challenging—to establish the international exchange of blood stem cells to save lives worldwide.

My involvement with transplants began more than 60 years ago when I had several jobs. One as the head of a blood bank and a second job as an internist interested in haematology and seeing patients with illnesses like leukaemia. At the same time, a colleague of mine, Dick van Bekkum, was busy developing a clinical protocol for bone marrow transplantation in mice and monkeys. We hoped with this approach, one day, we might cure radiation disease, leukaemia and other diseases of the blood-forming system.

Although Dick van Bekkum and I were following different paths, we were both pioneers—Dick van Bekkum with his experiments in laboratory animals and I with my investigations into blood transfusion medicine. We had our eyes open and saw an opportunity to help people. By coincidence we were living and studying in the same city. You might say we were in the right place, at the right time. Additionally, we were in a fortunate position financially because, at that time, the Dutch government was constructing the first nuclear reactors and establishing supportive facilities for researching radiation protection and treating victims of potential nuclear accidents. Among them were a specialised clinical ward at Leiden University Hospital that depended heavily on the blood bank, and a large, well-equipped Radiobiological Research Institute at nearby Rijswijk directed by Dick van Bekkum. By that time, the early 50s, it was known that exposure to high-dose radiation caused bone marrow failure. Blood transfusions were the only option, but did not result in a durable therapeutic effect, and bone marrow transplantation was still in its experimental stage in the laboratory.

I was working in what is now known as Leiden University Medical Centre. Initially we were far too busy taking care of patients who needed red blood cell (RBC) transfusions to worry about radiation accidents. The blood bank was a single room with two beds, two poorly trained lab technicians, a centrifuge you had to turn by hand, a microscope that required sunlight and a single refrigerator for storing the glass blood bottles. In the 1950s, blood banking was still in its early stages; the annual production of our blood bank was only about 4,000 bottles. But we were kept very busy because about 10 per cent of transfusions back then led to a non-haemolytic transfusion reaction (NHTR). This was an acute flu-like illness accompanied by a high fever, shaking chills, muscle

> "The cause was unknown until it was discovered that antibodies to white blood cells (WBCs) or leukocytes in transfusion recipients were responsible."

pain and sometimes hypotension, which could start a few hours after the blood had been transfused. The cause was unknown until

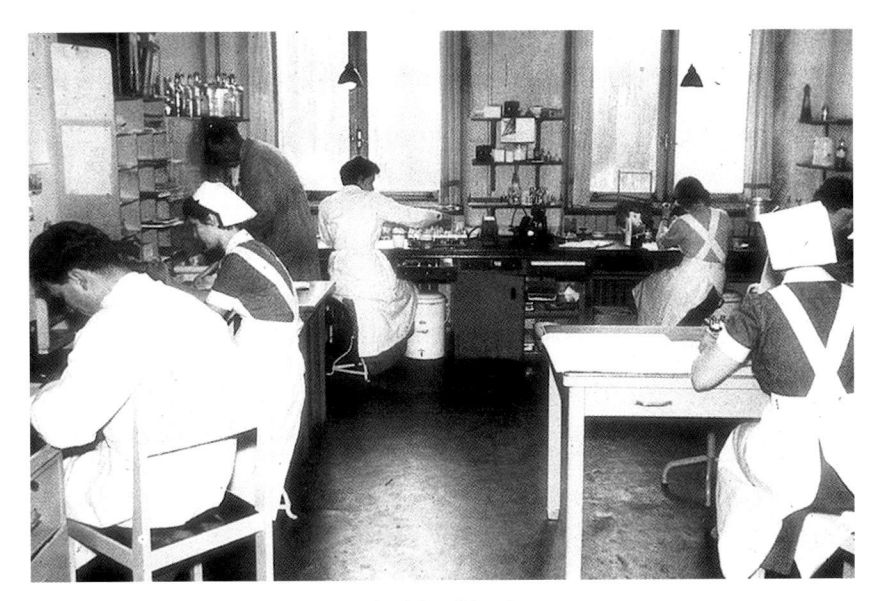

The blood bank

it was discovered that antibodies to white blood cells (WBCs) or leukocytes in transfusion recipients were responsible. At that time RBC transfusions contained white blood cells, whose function is to remove the broken down products of cells and bacteria. However, when white blood cells are destroyed by the recipient's antibodies, these bacterial remains enter the blood stream, causing an NHTR.

An NHTR is an unpleasant complication but, in general, is not dangerous. However, in individuals requiring frequent transfusions, e.g. for aplastic anaemia, these reactions become a nightmare. The logical solution was to remove the white blood cells from the transfusion—but there were no centrifuges for 500 ml bottles of blood! We improvised and were able to overcome the problem, to the great relief of our patients.

On 11 April 1958, I was called to the obstetrics department, where a woman who had delivered twins was bleeding heavily. She needed a red blood cell transfusion. A few hours later she developed a severe NHTR. She had lived in Leiden her whole life. She had never received a blood transfusion before! At that time, the general assumption of the experts was that antibodies to white blood cells were only formed following previous blood transfusions. This woman had never had a blood transfusion, but she had eight prior pregnancies. We realised that the experts might be wrong. We went to our serum freezer and found that roughly one in three pregnant women did indeed develop antibodies to white blood cells—findings that were soon confirmed by investigators in the US. This discovery had important implications. During a course on biostatistics, it became clear to me that the genetics of human leucocyte antigen (HLA), or of tissue groups recognised by these white blood cell antibodies, was extremely complex, and that we would need computers and statistics to unravel it.

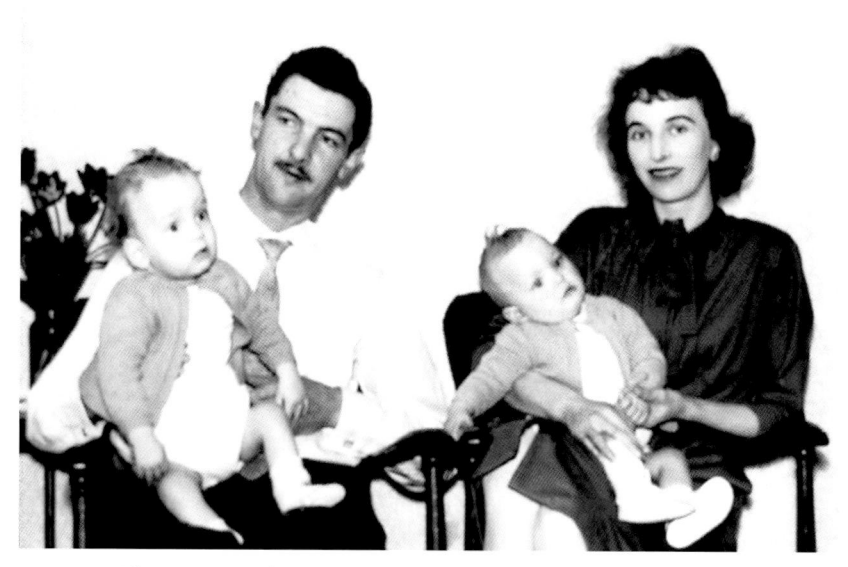

The woman whose pregnancy sparked the discovery of HLA.

Following this, we procured a new and better equipped laboratory and began studying the survival of red blood cells, white blood cells and platelets using radioisotopes. This work was led by George Eernisse, but everyone in the blood bank chipped in and helped. These studies taught us important lessons. For instance, I received so many experimental platelet transfusions that I made antibodies to white blood cells, which also turned out to react with platelets. We soon discovered that these antigens were present on the cells of all tissues and organs.

The study of white blood cells genetic markers had gone international by this point and was being funded by the US National Institutes of Health. These studies completed our understanding of the HLA system. The importance of HLA in transplantation was first proven in collaboration with Hans Balner, a physician in charge of the Primate Centre, at that time maintained by the Radiobiological Institute at Rijswijk. In those days it wasn't unusual to confirm findings in monkeys in human volunteers, and of course it was important to lead by example—so I and over a dozen other colleagues volunteered.

After much pre-clinical work we were prepared when, one day in 1968, Johan, a four-month-old baby suffering from immune system failure—severe combined immunodeficiency (SCID)—was admitted to the paediatrics clinic. Johan had severe skin and lung infections and was understandably miserable. But he was fortunate to have a sister who had the same tissue or HLA groups. Having SCID, Johan had an immediate advantage over children with leukaemia because there was no cancer that had to be eradicated. Johan was taken care of by the paediatricians Jaak Vossen, Han de Koning and Leo Jan Dooren, and became the recipient of the first long-term successful bone marrow transplant in Europe; Johan is still alive and I have seen him quite recently. Around the same time, two children underwent similarly successful stem cell transplants in the US; all three patients were subject to the stem cell transplantation protocol that Dick van Bekkum and his colleagues had shown to work well in monkeys.

> SCID is a group of inherited disorders that cause severe abnormalities of the immune system. These disorders lead to reduced or malfunctioning T- and B-lymphocytes, the specialised white blood cells made in the bone marrow and the thymus gland to fight infection. When the immune system doesn't function properly, it can be difficult or impossible for it to battle viruses, bacteria and fungi that cause infections.

Because of our success, Leiden became well known throughout Europe. People came from all over Europe for transplants, and many patients were cured. Despite this, the success rate remained at less than 50 per cent. Initially, bone marrow transplants were only performed in patients with a genetically identical twin or HLA-identical sibling. We soon realised that by doing an 'extended family search', more donors could be identified. The first recipient of this type of transplant was a patient suffering from immune deficiency, who travelled from Sicily to Leiden in 1971. His donor was an uncle, and the transplant was a success.

At this time the blood bank in Leiden also provided platelets. If a recipient had become immunised against the tissue or HLA groups, e.g. through previous blood transfusions or pregnancy, the platelets needed to be HLA-matched to prevent their destruction. Many blood donors were typed in order to find the best platelet donor for these recipients. We soon realised we could also help people who needed a bone marrow transplant but lacked an HLA identical or family donor. This led to the proposal in 1970 to launch Europdonor (the national unrelated donor registry of the Netherlands). The idea did not catch on at first, but eventually led to the first unrelated bone marrow transplant in a patient suffering from aplastic anaemia in Leiden in 1972. Since then the lives of countless people have been saved thanks to HLA-matched platelet transfusions and stem cell transplants with the support of volunteer donors.

Also in the 1970s, a haematologist called Bruno Speck came to Leiden from Switzerland. He had a particular interest in aplastic anaemia. After his arrival, we also turned our attention to treating different forms of leukaemia, following the protocols of the Nobel Prize Winner Dr Edward Donnall Thomas in the US. When we began transplanting leukaemia patients ourselves, the going was very rough. There were some awful complications—you can't imagine how poorly some of these patients were doing. It was also difficult for the nurses who were looking after the patients. At that time we did not have enough experience to know how to take good care of these patients.

After we had treated 10 patients, only one survived—which at that time was the 'success' rate other teams were experiencing as well. This patient was an Italian and was very homesick, so we sent him home. When he arrived back in Italy, his whole family was there to greet him. They were so pleased to see him that they kissed him all over. As a result of that, he caught a virus and sadly passed away. So these were very difficult times. After postponing our transplantation work for a while, a new team was brought in and a better protocol established, which offered much improved chances of survival.

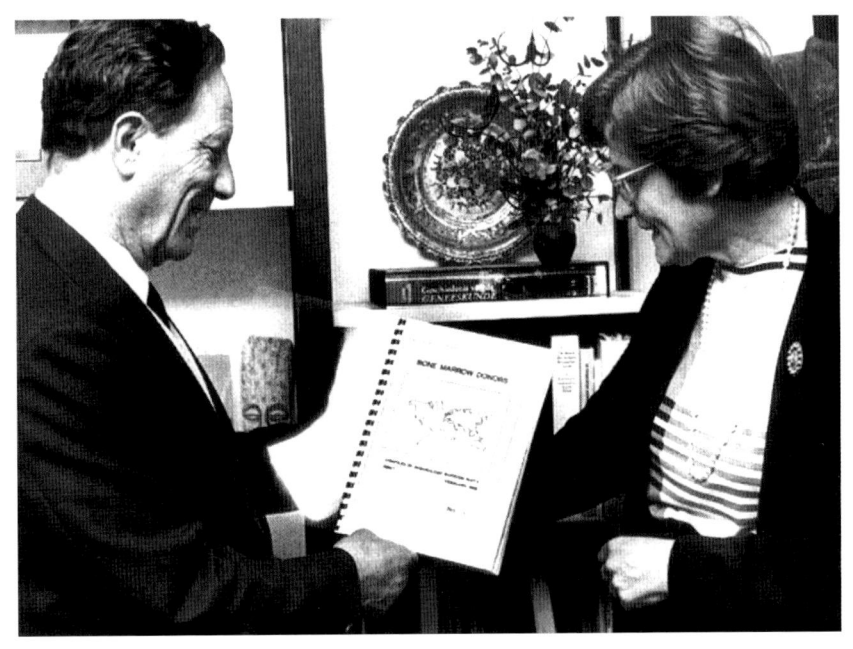

Jon (left) and Aad holding the first edition of BMDW.

It wasn't until 1980 that the first successful unrelated transplants to treat leukaemia took place in the US. I remember going to conferences and meeting other doctors, and the question we would ask one another was, "How many of your patients are still alive after

In the right place, at the right time

three months?" As time went on, there were more and more people who had one, two or even three patients who had survived the procedure. After a while, we too had more patients who survived. It was really good to see how they returned to their lives. However, the follow-up was not always so favourable—and sometimes it still isn't today. I remember a girl with acute myeloid leukaemia who received a transplant using stem cells from her father. The transplant was successful and she was cured of her leukaemia, but as a result she developed chronic graft-versus-host disease, which made her skin dry and painful. When she visited me at the hospital, she told me that her boyfriend had ended their relationship. She ended by saying: "I sometimes wish that you hadn't performed the transplant."

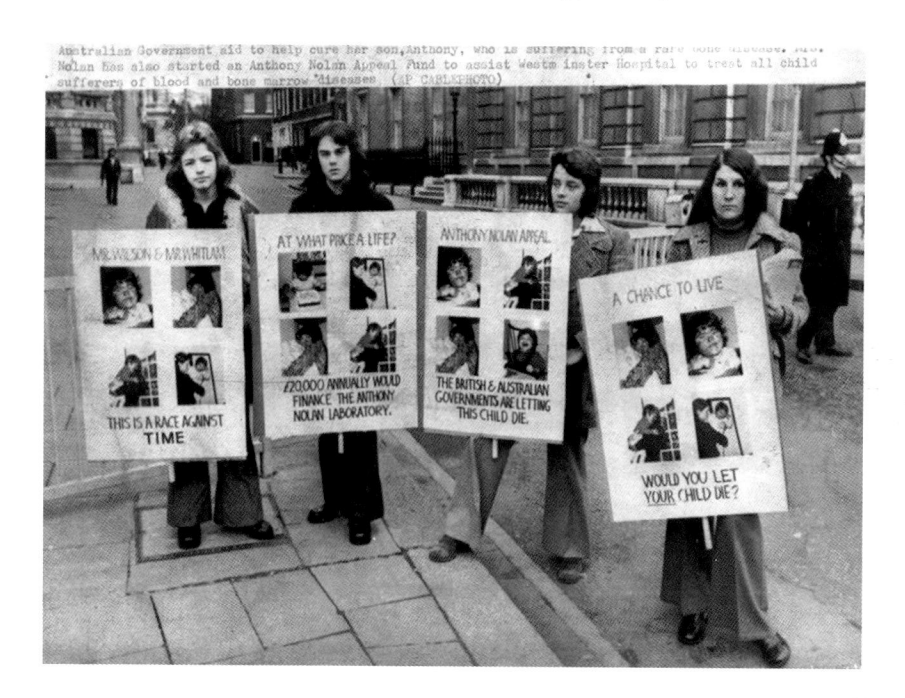

The next hurdle we faced was that the HLA system is extremely complex and polymorphic, which meant that many donors were needed in order to find a match. Fortunately, Shirley Nolan had also started a bone marrow donor registry of volunteer adult donors in 1974 in the United Kingdom. We worked closely together from the beginning, and I sent HLA typing reagents to London when they organised a donor drive. In the late 1980s, the US and five other countries in Europe also launched their own bone marrow donor registry. However, the idea that we should work together and exchange stem cells between different countries was not generally accepted. To add to the problem, we were only able to communicate using post, telephone and fax—Internet was not yet available, and hence finding a matched donor in another country was quite time consuming. After much discussion, the idea of collecting the HLA groups of all volunteers of the eight registries active at that time was accepted by all, and Bone Marrow Donors Worldwide (BMDW), a database containing the HLA or tissue groups of all volunteer stem cell donors in the world was born. All new registries joined the effort, and today BMDW is consulted around 200,000 times a year.

The BMDW has also been an important source of genetic information. Once we had two million donors on file, we noticed that a sizeable proportion had an HLA group that occurred only once. These people had a unique HLA group. The crucial question was: how do we help patients with a unique HLA group? It was clear that we needed more donors! So that became our focus. Today we have more than 25 million volunteer donors who are willing to help any patient in need of a transplant.

To further complicate matters, the complexity of HLA in India or South America is quite different from that in Europe. That's because this complexity also has a biological function. It's important to understand that the role of HLA is not to frustrate patients and their doctors—it is to protect people from infections that are common in the part of the world where they live. This means you cannot help European patients with donors from Africa or South America. We soon realised that *finding* a suitable donor was one problem we could resolve with BMDW—but that if we really wanted to help patients, we had to organise the *international transfer* of stem cells. Sending stem cells to another country in the late 1980s presented a whole host of challenges: from the problems of trying to physically pass through customs with the containers, to costs related to health insurance.

> "Sending stem cells to another country in the late 1980s presented a whole host of challenges: from the problems of trying to physically pass through customs with the containers, to costs related to health insurance."

The late John Goldman, who was in charge of Anthony Nolan at that time, was already a figure of great authority and was well respected in our field. One day, at a conference in Keystone near Denver, US, he brought together a small group of doctors in a very nice room overlooking the ski slopes. The issue at hand was how to organise the exchange of stem cells between different countries—not only the legal side of it, but also in terms of customs, insurance, and medical and ethical aspects. Everyone agreed that something had to be done, and as a result of that discussion, a paper was published that contained a rough outline of what is now the mission of the World Marrow Donor Association (WMDA)*.

Later on, in 1988, the same group was to have a meeting in Düsseldorf, Germany. More and more people were showing an interest in WMDA. I met John Goldman shortly before the meeting and he told me that he was considering cancelling it because he had other commitments. That was around the time he was starting the scientific journal Bone Marrow Transplantation, so he was very busy. I pointed out that some people had travelled all the way from the US to attend the meeting, and had even paid for their own tickets. I said, "John, I understand you're busy, but we cannot cancel this meeting."

So I offered to chair the meeting myself. John's response was typical, "Please do take over, Jon, I have too many fiddles to play."

At our next meeting in Vienna, I realised—while listening to Susan Cleaver from Anthony Nolan in particular—that if we really wanted to get the WMDA working, it had to be better organised. I therefore came up with a pyramid structure. At the bottom, we had the working groups who would be manned by people like Susan, whose day-to-day role was finding donors. And then, we had representatives from the various regions: the Americas, Asia, Oceania and Europe. Finally there was the President, which at that time was me. John Goldman took up the post of Secretary General.

The history of the WMDA has shown that we needed this kind of global forum to determine what we can and cannot ask of our volunteer donors. One very important thing to remember is that transplantation is not over once a donor has donated—not only for the patient, but for the donor too. Some countries, like the US, give their donors updates on patients after their transplant—and some donors find it very difficult if they learn that their 'gift of life' wasn't successful. So that's another aspect of the WMDA's role. I'm certain that the WMDA will continue to play an extremely important role for a very long time to come, especially if it can continue to act with speed and flexibility in the rapidly changing world of stem cell transplants.

*Special report: Bone marrow transplants using volunteer donors—recommendations and requirements for a standardized practice throughout the world (Bone Marrow Transplantation, 1992, 10: 287-291).

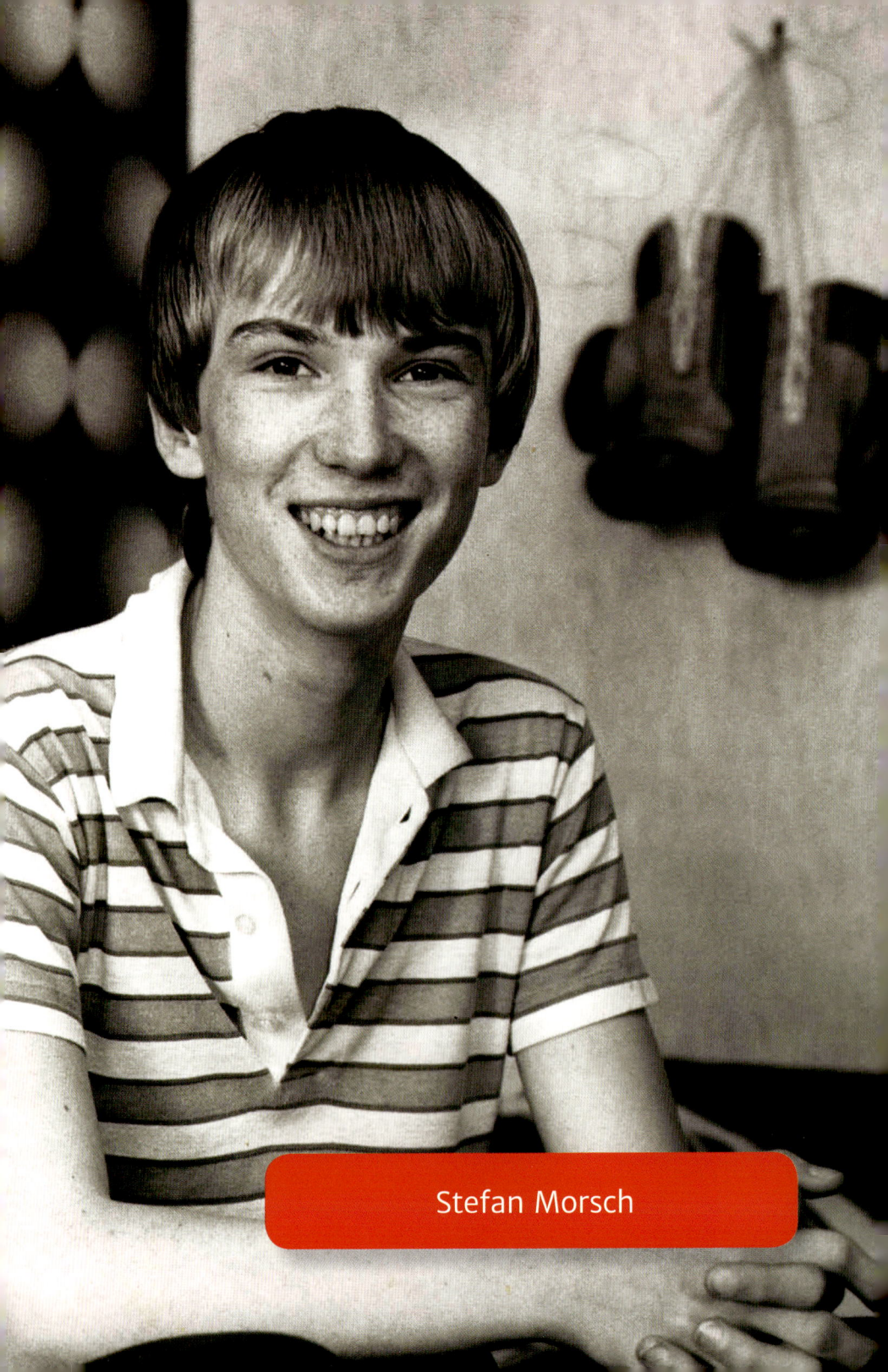

Stefan Morsch

Proud

Susanne Morsch, Search Coordinator at the Stefan Morsch Foundation, Germany

I was eight years younger than my brother Stefan, but we were very close. When we were young, we enjoyed playing football together, climbing trees and even playing tricks on our parents! I had the best older brother any little girl could hope for. But when Stefan was just 16, our family's world was turned upside down.

One day, Stefan came home complaining of bad stomach pains. Our family doctor suspected appendicitis and ordered some blood tests. But when the results came back, he broke the devastating news to my family that everything pointed towards leukaemia. He recommended that my brother be admitted to the hospital immediately.

After further tests, we learned that my brother was suffering from chronic myeloid leukaemia. Unfortunately, medication and chemotherapy alone would not be enough to save Stefan, so the hospital recommended a stem cell transplant. Each member of our family was HLA-typed in the hope of finding a suitable donor. I remember being very excited as I was sure that I would be a match for my brother. Our family was confident that my brother would be treated successfully and return home healthy.

However, test results revealed that no match had been found in our family. We were heartbroken. The doctors told my parents that without a donor and transplant, nothing more could be done for Stefan. All they could do was to administer treatment to Stefan that would prolong his life without curing his leukaemia. They suggested that we focus on making what was left of his life as enjoyable and comfortable as possible.

> Chronic myeloid leukaemia (CML) is a type of blood cancer where a switch of genes between two different chromosomes results in a mutated white blood cell that grows too fast. Bone marrow transplants used to be the best method for treating and curing these patients. Nowadays, some new drugs can be given to treat and bring this disease into complete remission, a state where cancer cells can no longer be detected, though it may not mean that all cancer cells have been eliminated. It is not currently known whether these new drugs can be stopped when a patient is in complete remission, so a bone marrow transplant remains the only cure—especially for patients who have developed relapsed or more aggressive forms of CML.

But my parents did not give up. They did everything they could to make sure Stefan lived his life like any healthy teenager, including attending his favourite team's football games and going on holidays. At the same time, they kept on searching for another way to save his life.

Finally, in July 1983, my dad came across an article about an eight-year-old child who had undergone a bone marrow transplant in London, thanks to Nolan Laboratories, which is now called Anthony Nolan. At that time, they had a register of 50,000 volunteer donors. Doctors in Germany told us that a transplant using an unrelated donor was considered an experimental treatment. It had never been done in Europe before. But for our family, it was a glimmer of hope.

Dad contacted Anthony Nolan and the search for an unrelated bone marrow donor began. There was only a one in 700,000 chance of finding a potential donor, but Anthony Nolan identified 94 potential stem cell donors whose tissue typing matched Stefan's in three of the four factors considered critical for acceptance at that time. Finally, a donor was identified: Terence Bayley. Terence was married and had a little boy, with a second child on the way. More importantly, he was ready and willing to donate his stem cells.

The next challenge was to find a hospital that would be willing to help us save Stefan. Anthony Nolan suggested that we look in the US. And sure enough, a team led by one of the founders of the WMDA, Dr Edward Donnall Thomas from the Fred Hutchinson Cancer Research Center in Seattle, agreed to perform the transplant.

A few days before Stefan and my parents were scheduled to fly to Seattle, we encountered another setback. There was no insurance that would cover the potential risks for the donor, which meant that my parents had to come up with a security deposit. Our family's savings had already been depleted paying for the flights and treatment.

We were out of ideas. Fortunately, our local mayor was not. He knew about our situation, so he contacted the media and launched a charity appeal.

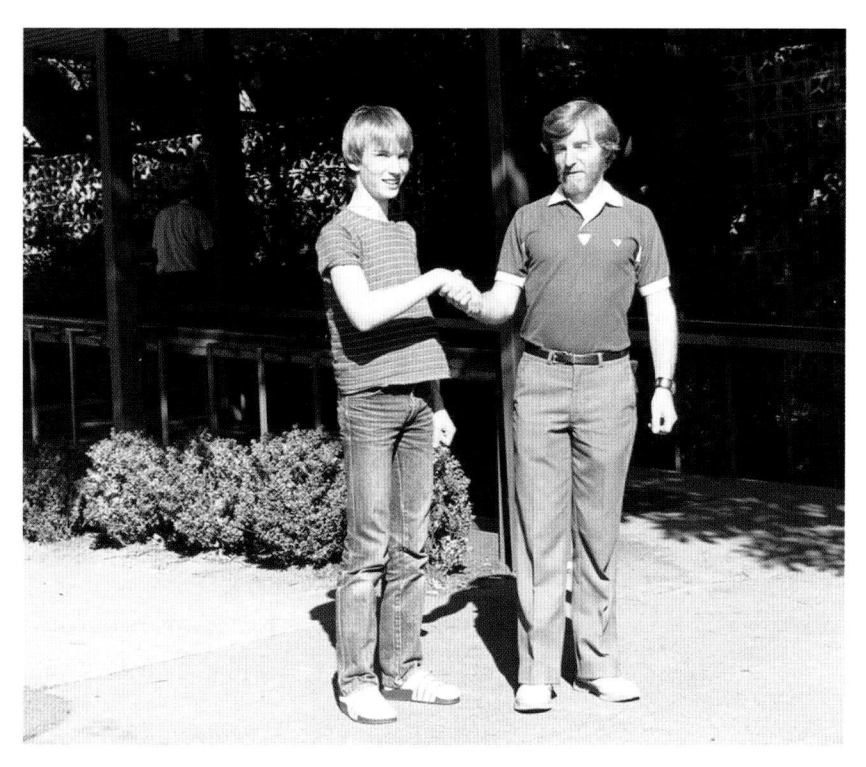

Stefan had an opportunity to meet his donor, Terence Bayley.

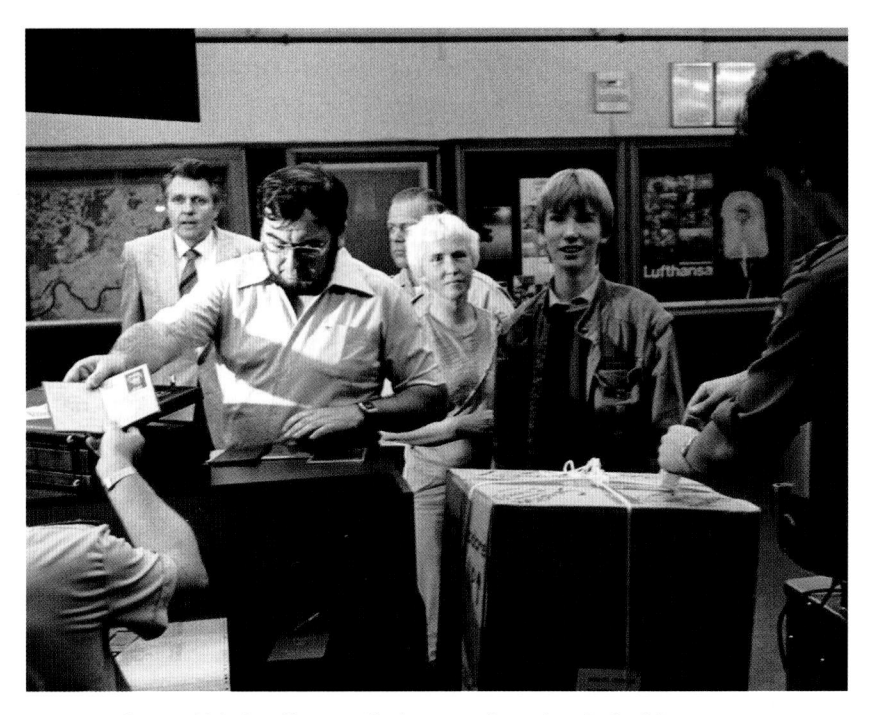

Stefan and his family travelled across the Atlantic for his treatment.

Within a couple of days, people had donated the equivalent of more than 400,000 euros to save Stefan, which meant that my family could finally travel to the US.

In Seattle, Stefan came face-to-face with his donor, Terence. Both underwent extensive medical checks and on 31 July 1984, Stefan underwent the transplant. The next day, Terence sat beside Stefan's isolation tent, watching him sleep and writing him a letter before he returned to his family in the UK.

During his time in hospital, Stefan received hundreds of letters from people all over the world—from family and friends, as well as complete strangers. Their good wishes were appreciated, but Stefan's condition fluctuated. One day he would feel better, but the next day he would suffer from a severe fever, chills and shakes. The long search for a donor and the treatment had weakened Stefan's body, and he had to fight a number of infections. Because the medical team did not have very much experience with unrelated transplants, no one really knew what to expect.

As Christmas approached, Stefan's condition started to improve and he was discharged from the hospital. Preparations were made for his return to Germany so that we could all celebrate Christmas at home together. My dad flew back to Seattle to help out, but by that point Stefan had fallen ill again—with chickenpox, for the second time. While Stefan's weakened body was fighting the virus, the next complication came along—pneumonia.

When my parents arrived at the hospital on 17 December, they were told that Stefan's lungs had started to fill with water. They sat down and Stefan rested his head in my mother's arms. After a while, he fell asleep. Then his heart simply stopped beating.

Although Stefan lost the fight for his life, he did not lose the fight against leukaemia. It was his wish to set up a stem cell donor registry in Germany to give other leukaemia patients a second chance at life.

> "Although Stefan lost the fight for his life, he did not lose the fight against leukaemia. It was his wish to set up a stem cell donor registry in Germany to give other leukaemia patients a second chance at life."

While Stefan was in hospital, our family had been contacted by many other patients and their families. After he passed away, the number of calls increased. We pointed them towards Anthony Nolan for help in their search for donors and to the hospital in Seattle for the transplant. This support eventually led to the establishment of the Stefan Morsch Foundation, which was launched using funds that had been donated to finance Stefan's treatment.

In the following years, more and more German organisations began to emerge and it became clear to my parents that a centralised database of German patients and donors was needed. With financial backing from the Stefan Morsch Foundation, a central registry for Germany was established in May 1992: the German National Registry of Blood Stem Cell Donors (ZKRD).

Looking back on everything that has happened since Stefan's death, I feel very proud. I am proud of my parents for turning such a tragic

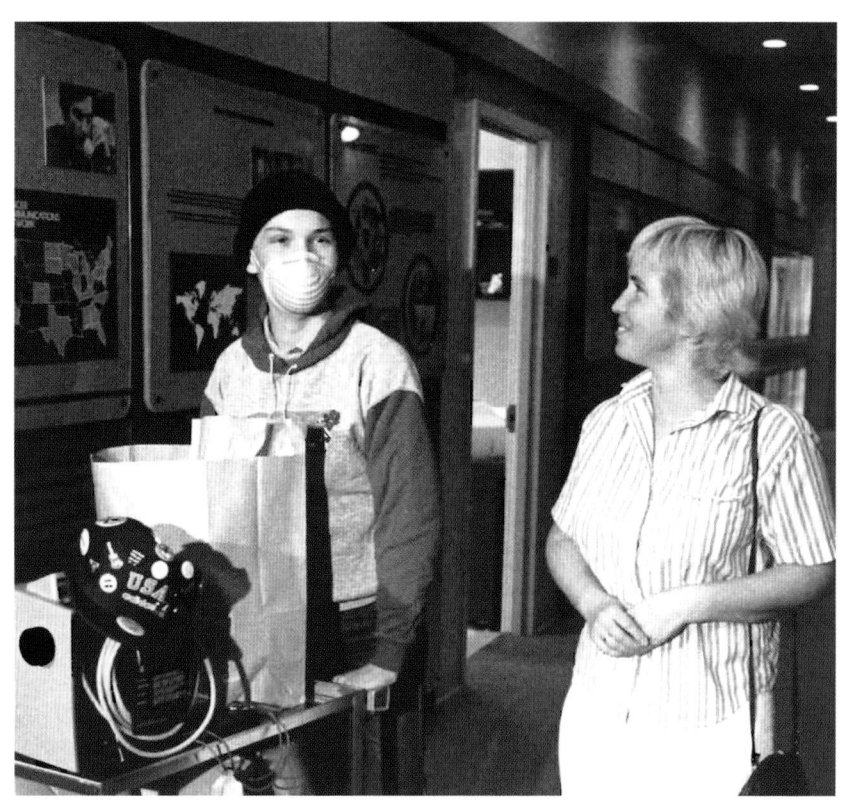

Stefan leaving the hospital.

event into something so meaningful. I am proud of our team at the Stefan Morsch Foundation, who work so very hard to recruit donors and to help patients. I am proud of all the unrelated stem cell donors who have stepped up to save a stranger's life. Most of all, I am proud of my brother who was a true fighter and who taught me never to give up. I know that he would also be proud of what the Foundation has achieved in his name.

SSDS WALKS FOR LIFE IN SUPPORT OF JAY FEINBER

Miracle match

Jay Feinberg, recipient of a bone marrow transplant in 1995

I was 23 years old and fresh out of college. I was working in New York as a financial analyst and had just been accepted into law school; I felt as though I was ready to take on the world. Life was good.

All that changed quickly one day when I went to the family doctor for what I thought was a case of the flu. He performed a blood count and, before I knew it, he sent me to the emergency room at my local hospital. My life was about to change forever.

I was frightened when the doctor at the hospital told me I had leukaemia, but felt reassured when I learnt that a stem cell transplant could save my life. At least I had a chance.

We scheduled an appointment at a large hospital near my home and on that day my mother, father, two brothers and I all crammed into the small examination room to hear the news. It was not good. My brothers were not matches and no matched donor had been found in the international database of stem cell donors. The doctor added, "It is highly unlikely you will ever find a match due to your rare tissue type and ethnicity. You see, Jews are under-represented in the worldwide donor pool—it's like looking for a needle in a haystack."

I had no idea then that tissue type was inherited in the same way as eye or hair colour, or that a patient's best chance of finding a genetic match was with someone of similar ethnic origin. The doctor started me on chemotherapy, and encouraged me to go home and do all the things I wanted to do—to prepare my bucket list and enjoy life while I could.

But that was not my destiny. You see, my mother, Arlene, was the quintessential mother. She would not take no for an answer, and was not going to sit by and watch her son die. That was how the 'Friends of Jay' bone marrow recruitment campaign began. It all started at my parents' dining room table. We began preparing flyers with headlines such as 'Urgent appeal. Please don't let me die.' It was not easy being the poster child of this hard-hitting campaign, but we did what we had to do.

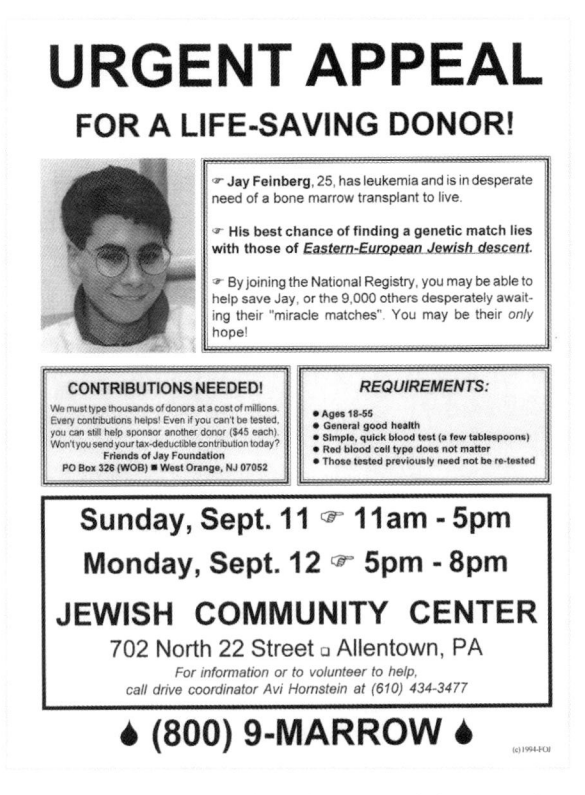

URGENT APPEAL
FOR A LIFE-SAVING DONOR!

- Jay Feinberg, 25, has leukemia and is in desperate need of a bone marrow transplant to live.
- His best chance of finding a genetic match lies with those of *Eastern-European Jewish descent*.
- By joining the National Registry, you may be able to help save Jay, or the 9,000 others desperately awaiting their "miracle matches". You may be their *only* hope!

CONTRIBUTIONS NEEDED!
We must type thousands of donors at a cost of millions. Every contribution helps! Even if you can't be tested, you can still help sponsor another donor ($45 each). Won't you send your tax-deductible contribution today?
Friends of Jay Foundation
PO Box 326 (WOB) ■ West Orange, NJ 07052

REQUIREMENTS:
- Ages 18-55
- General good health
- Simple, quick blood test (a few tablespoons)
- Red blood cell type does not matter
- Those tested previously need not be re-tested

Sunday, Sept. 11 ☞ 11am - 5pm
Monday, Sept. 12 ☞ 5pm - 8pm
JEWISH COMMUNITY CENTER
702 North 22 Street □ Allentown, PA
For information or to volunteer to help,
call drive coordinator Avi Hornstein at (610) 434-3477

♦ **(800) 9-MARROW** ♦

The urgent appeal flyer that started the campaign.

We hosted our first donor drive at our local synagogue. The response was unexpected and emotionally overwhelming. Crowds of people appeared and the line to get tested snaked out the door, extending into the parking lot. There were hundreds of people who cared enough to save the life of a total stranger. It was awe-inspiring.

Soon after, calls started to pour in from New York, California, Connecticut, Israel, Canada and Australia. Callers had seen stories in the media about my public search for a donor and they wanted to help. A movement had begun.

Throughout my donor search and treatment for leukaemia, it was the incredible response from the public that kept me going. Before we knew it, we were working out of 2,000 square feet of donated office space with a team of dedicated volunteers, orchestrating drives all over the US and worldwide. Yet this journey was never just about me. My mother became the consummate patient advocate— helping other families in similar circumstances, guiding them along the right path and sharing her knowledge. Day and night, weekdays and weekends, she was on the phone, giving patients and families comfort in their time of need.

Four years later, my disease had accelerated. Chemotherapy was no longer keeping me in the chronic phase and my time was drawing near. I prepared for a transplant with a donor who was a multiple mismatch. It was risky but it was my only chance. I made my way to Seattle, where I would receive my transplant at the Fred Hutchinson Cancer Research Center.

It was then that a young man from Chicago contacted my family. His name was Benji and he wanted to help me find my match because a Friends of Jay drive had found a match for his close friend in Toronto. How could we say no? Even though I was preparing for my transplant with a less than optimal match, at least his drive could help others in need. So we gave him the green light to proceed.

The drive took place on a beautiful spring day at a yeshiva in Milwaukee. Towards the end of the drive, a volunteer named Becky stretched out her arm to donate a sample of blood. After four years, 225 donor drives and 60,000 donors, that young lady turned out to be my match —my miracle match. She saved my life!

A year later, as I disembarked from a flight to Chicago, a crowd greeted me at the gate. It was Becky and her family. We cried and embraced as we greeted each other for the very first time. I will never forget that day or my week-long visit with Becky and her wonderful family.

Shortly after I returned home to New Jersey, the phone rang. It was the dean at the law school where I had been accepted. It turned out that he had held my place for five years and followed my donor search closely. He knew about my transplant and invited me back to law school! I thanked him for his kindness, but told him that my life now had new meaning and was taking me in a different direction. I wanted to give back for the gift I had received. I wanted to grow the incredible resource my family and friends had built and help those in similar circumstances. He understood. And so, Friends of Jay became 'Gift of Life'. The rest, as they say, is history.

> "I wanted to give back for the gift I had received. I wanted to grow the incredible resource my family and friends had built and help those in similar circumstances. He understood. And so, Friends of Jay became 'Gift of Life'. The rest, as they say, is history."

I made it my mission to help find a match for any patient in need, whenever they needed one. And I had learned a lot over the preceding six years to help me—about tissue typing, family studies, unrelated donor searches and so much more. I thank John Hansen, Paul Martin and Lori Hubbard at the Fred Hutchinson Cancer Research Center for that education; it has been invaluable.

When we founded Gift of Life, my family's vision was that no patient should die for lack of a donor and that no family should have to go through what we endured. This remains our guiding principle to this day. With a passionate and dedicated team of nearly 50 employees and more than 2,000 volunteers, Gift of Life is nearly a quarter of a million donors strong.

We value quality, efficiency and innovation. We were the first registry to implement buccal swabs at donor drives, the first with an online registration system giving people the ability to swab at home and much more. We are always seeking ways to improve ourselves for the benefit of patients. And we will continue to advance the cause and work closely with all the global registries until our vision becomes a reality.

Through this journey, I have learned that one person can make a difference. Whether it is a donor joining the registry at a drive, an advocate comforting a patient in need, or a cancer survivor choosing to give back for his or her second chance at life—the power of the individual is undeniable.

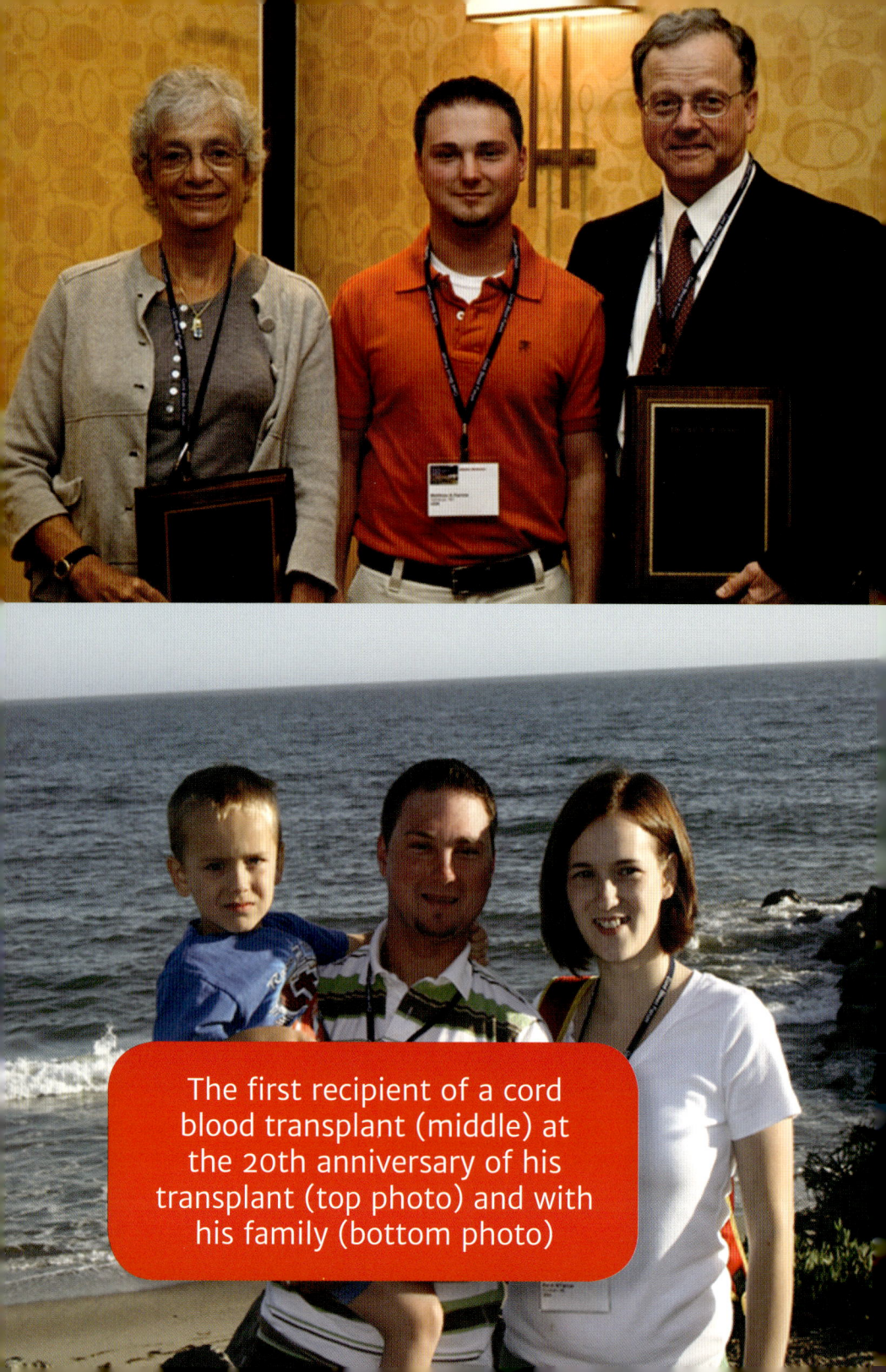

The first recipient of a cord blood transplant (middle) at the 20th anniversary of his transplant (top photo) and with his family (bottom photo)

Blazing trails in cord blood transplantation

Prof Eliane Gluckman, Director of Eurocord, President of the European School of Haematology and Head of the International Sickle Cell Disease Observatory

I became head of the bone marrow transplant unit at Saint-Louis Hospital in Paris in 1973. The unit was the first of its kind in Europe. Prior to this, I had gained many years' experience training in bone marrow transplantation and haematology in both the US and France. At Saint-Louis, I began to focus more on non-malignant diseases in children because it was a paediatrics unit as well.

This was what led me to perform the first ever cord blood transplant in 1988. I had been working on sickle cell transplantation beforehand, as well as on the conditioning of Fanconi's anaemia patients, so I had a strong background in this area.

> Fanconi's anaemia is a rare, inherited disease that leads to aplastic anaemia. Children born with it tend to be smaller than average and have birth defects such as underdeveloped limbs. Aplastic anaemia is a condition that occurs when your body stops producing enough new blood cells.

The first cord blood transplantation in 1988 was very successful. Unlike most cord blood transplants, the donor in this instance was

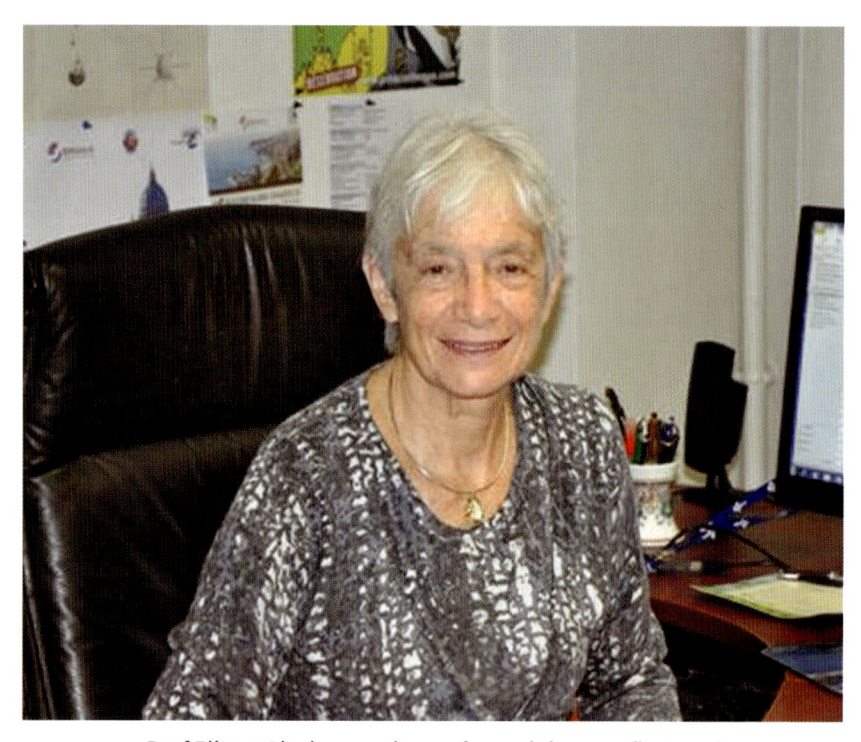

Prof Eliane Gluckman who performed the very first cord blood transplant in 1988.

an HLA-identical sibling—the patient's sister. Although he was just five years old at the time, the patient had a prompt donor engraftment and did not suffer any complications. He is now more than 25 years post-transplant and is completely cured.

I still hear from the patient often. In fact, I saw him on the 20th anniversary of his transplant. That was quite a celebration. It was very interesting to hear him talk about his life now and how little he remembers of the transplant. When I meet patients who have received a cord blood transplant, and who would probably have died without it, it is extremely rewarding.

Since that transplant, we have gone on to set up a global network of cord blood banks. Now there are more than 600,000 cord blood units stored in public cord blood banks all over the world. At Eurocord we keep a registry of cord blood transplants, and so far we have been able to collect data on at least 30,000. We track them and analyse the data so that we can propose new ways of using these cells.

The benefit of cord blood transplantation over other types of stem cell transplants is that you can collect the blood in advance, test it for infectious disease markers and then cryopreserve it. Cord blood can be stored in banks forever, so if there is an emergency and you need a transplant immediately, the cord blood is readily available.

Another key advantage is that the immune systems of newborns are immature, which means there are very few immunological reactions post-transplant. This is the main benefit of non-HLA identical transplants.

Nowadays approximately 20 per cent of transplants use cord blood, but it really depends on the preference of the individual hospital or medical centre. To donate your baby's cord blood, you need to be in a maternity unit that is accredited for collection. Some private banks have tried to sell the idea of donating cord blood for your own use, but at Eurocord we do not recommend that.

> "Now there are more than 600,000 cord blood units stored in public cord blood banks all over the world."

There are many people who would like to donate their baby's cord blood, but what we need now is for more hospitals to become certified as cord blood collection centres. We probably only use about 10 per cent of the cord blood that is harvested as the quality of the blood is very important—so selecting the best cases is a lot of work. But all this work is worth it once you see the number of lives that are saved.

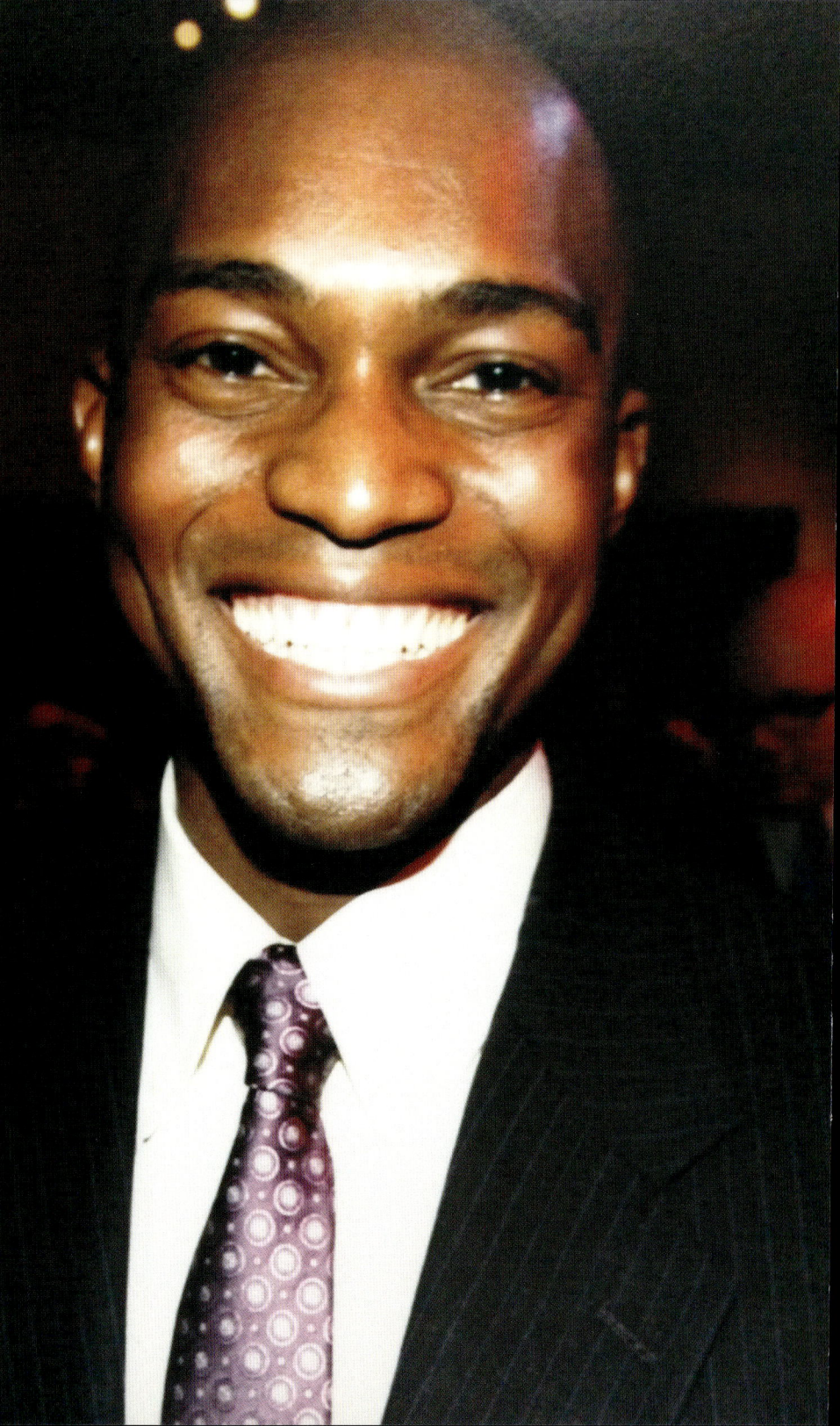

Planting a seed

Seun Adebiyi, recipient of a bone marrow transplant in 2010

It is a bleak, wintry afternoon in Manhattan. I glance nervously at the clock on the wall in the transplant suite. My consultation is scheduled to begin at any moment, but another two hours passed before the head transplant physician at Memorial Sloan Kettering strides into the room and launches into rapid-fire speech. As she speaks, my heart thumps against my ribcage with alternating beats of dread ... hope ... and dread.

After six months of searching, I still have not found a matching donor for a bone marrow transplant. My best odds of finding a donor lie within my own ethnic group, so in a few hours I am flying to Nigeria to host the country's first-ever bone marrow donor drive. However, there has been a change in plans.

A cord blood unit has just been located with cord blood from a Nigerian mother who gave birth in the US. I will have a transplant after all! However, international travel could jeopardise my transplant by exposing me to health risks like influenza and malaria. My doctor urges me to cancel my trip, go home and stay out of harm's way until my transplant is over.

My elation fades as quickly as it bloomed. Every day, thousands of black patients fruitlessly search the international registries for a matching donor. In the US, less than 17 per cent of black patients find a matched donor. In Africa, the situation is even worse. Millions of Nigerians suffer from blood disorders—such as sickle-cell anaemia—which can be successfully treated through bone marrow transplantation. South Africa is currently the only country on the continent with a fully operational donor registry; however, its donors are predominantly Caucasian.

With over 170 million people and 250 ethnic groups, the sheer size and diversity of Nigeria's population make it an ideal location for a new registry. I know that holding a donor drive in Nigeria is the first step to creating that registry, so with apprehension (and against doctor's orders), I board a plane to Lagos. Two days later, almost 300 Nigerians join the international donor community.

Two years later, the Bone Marrow Registry in Nigeria (BMRN)—the first donor registry in Nigeria and only the second in Africa—opens its doors at the University of Nigeria in Nnsuka. Its mission is to improve access to genetically diverse stem cell donors from Nigeria and to match patients all over the world with life-saving stem cell donors. To date, the BMRN has received search requests from 14 countries, with a 40 per cent match rate. Approximately 70 per cent of the search requests are from outside Nigeria.

> "Had my donor given birth in Nigeria instead of America, I might not be alive today—because there is still no public cord blood bank in Africa."

Five years later, thanks to my cord blood transplant, I continue to enjoy full remission from cancer. I am using my second chance at life to create more birthdays for others as a project manager for the American Cancer Society. Had my donor given birth in Nigeria instead of America, I might not be alive today—because there is still no public cord blood bank in Africa. The potential impact of closing this infrastructure gap is mind-boggling. According to one study, 40,000 cord blood units could save as many patients of African descent as a bone marrow registry of four million adults.

I hope that readers of this book will better appreciate the value of collaborating with African institutions to help patients around the world. Much more can—and should—be done to close the disparity between the chances of survival for white and black transplant candidates. A person's chance of surviving cancer should not be determined by their race or ethnicity.

Recruiting unique genetics

Dr Amal Bishara, Arab Donor Project, based in Jerusalem

In memory of Nur

We launched the Arab Donor Project in October 2008. The speech I gave to medical staff and the media to announce the launch of the project was dedicated to one of our patients: a young boy called Nur. Sadly, Nur had passed away from a genetic blood disease just 10 days before this very important event. I still remember how the lecture room fell silent when I announced that he had passed away because we could not find a matched donor in time.

Nur was the second child of a family from the West Bank. His older sibling also died at a very young age, most likely due to the same genetic disease. Nur also had a one-year-old sister, Limar, who was diagnosed with the same life-threatening disease just a few weeks after Nur passed away.

A donor could not be found for Limar in either the local or international registries, so the family decided to have another baby in the hope of saving their daughter. The pregnancy went smoothly and, after a DNA sample had been obtained and HLA typing performed, the baby was found to be a 10/10 match. The baby's cord blood was collected and later infused into the veins of Nur's sister. Although her recovery was slow, Limar was saved. Now she is healthy and beautiful, with the same deep green eyes that Nur had.

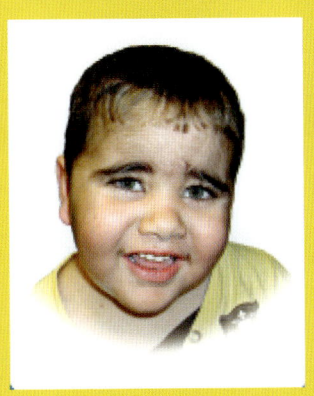

Baby Muhammad

Muhammad was just three months old in August 2010 when we received a donor search request for him. His family had already suffered one tragedy: their first son, Mahmoud, had suffered from the same disease and had died of complications, as no suitable stem cell donor could be found for him in the international database. This made our search for a donor for baby Muhammad even more critical.

The only matched donor we could identify was very young—an 18-year-old called Mahran who had registered as a volunteer donor just a few months earlier. After the collection of his stem cells, Mahran called me every few months to ask about the patient's recovery. I told him as much as I knew—that baby Muhammad had been engrafted and was doing okay, but was not gaining weight.

Then, a few weeks before the anniversary of the transplant, Mahran asked me to set up a meeting between him, Muhammad and Muhammad's family. They agreed.

I was very excited to organise our first donor/recipient meeting since the launch

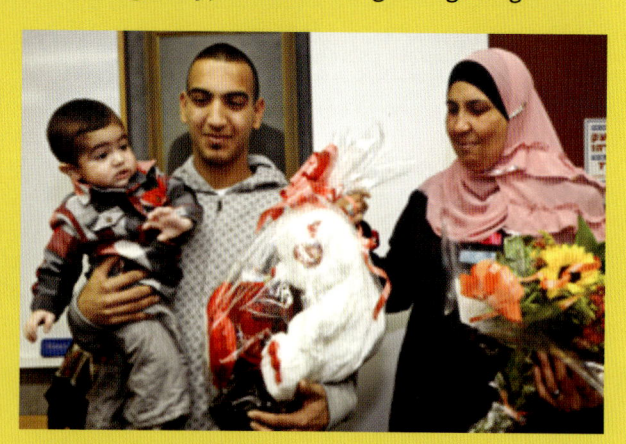

Donor Mahran is still in contact with Muhammad and his family.

of our Arab Donor Project in 2008, as were all my colleagues at the Hadassah registry. When the day came, I went to meet Muhammad and his family at the hospital and could hardly believe my eyes. Baby Muhammad looked the picture of health and had a big smile on his face. Now he's almost four years old and Mahran calls him 'little brother'. They still meet occasionally.

Hala

After a long and frustrating search for a matched donor for four-year-old Hala, we finally found one: a 40-year-old man from a village in the Galilee region. Muhammad was very cooperative from the first moment we made contact. The request from the girl's medical team was for bone marrow donation only, and he agreed. On the day of the donation, Muhammad arrived alone. I spent some time speaking with him and learned that he had two daughters, one of whom was the same age as the patient. The procedure ran very smoothly and Muhammad's recovery was extremely fast. Within just a few days he had returned to work, which was all the more impressive given that he worked in construction!

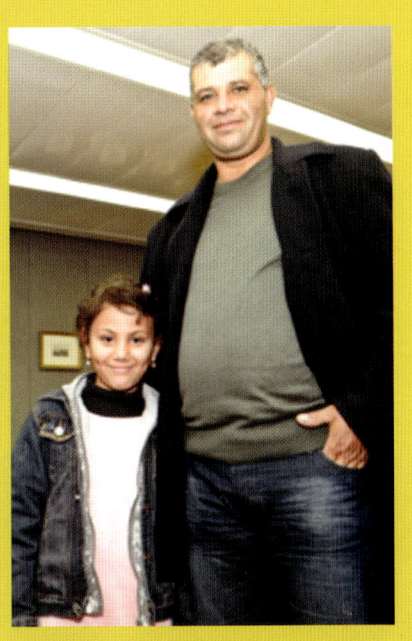

Muhammad with Hala, the young girl whose life he saved. Both families still meet regularly.

Afterwards, Muhammad called regularly to ask about the patient's recovery, and eventually we were able to organise a meeting between him and the patient's family. On the day of the meeting, Hala and her family came to the Hadassah Medical Centre in Jerusalem. Both families were very excited and emotional, and Muhammad's daughters presented Hala with a few small gifts.

> Finding a suitable donor for a stem cell transplant means finding a donor whose HLA tissue type matches that of the patient. Because HLA types are inherited, patients often find their most suitable donors within their own ethnic groups, even if the donor is from another country. Therefore, to give patients the best chance of finding a match for transplantation, it is important that registries recruit donors from various ethnic groups.

Recruiting unique genetics

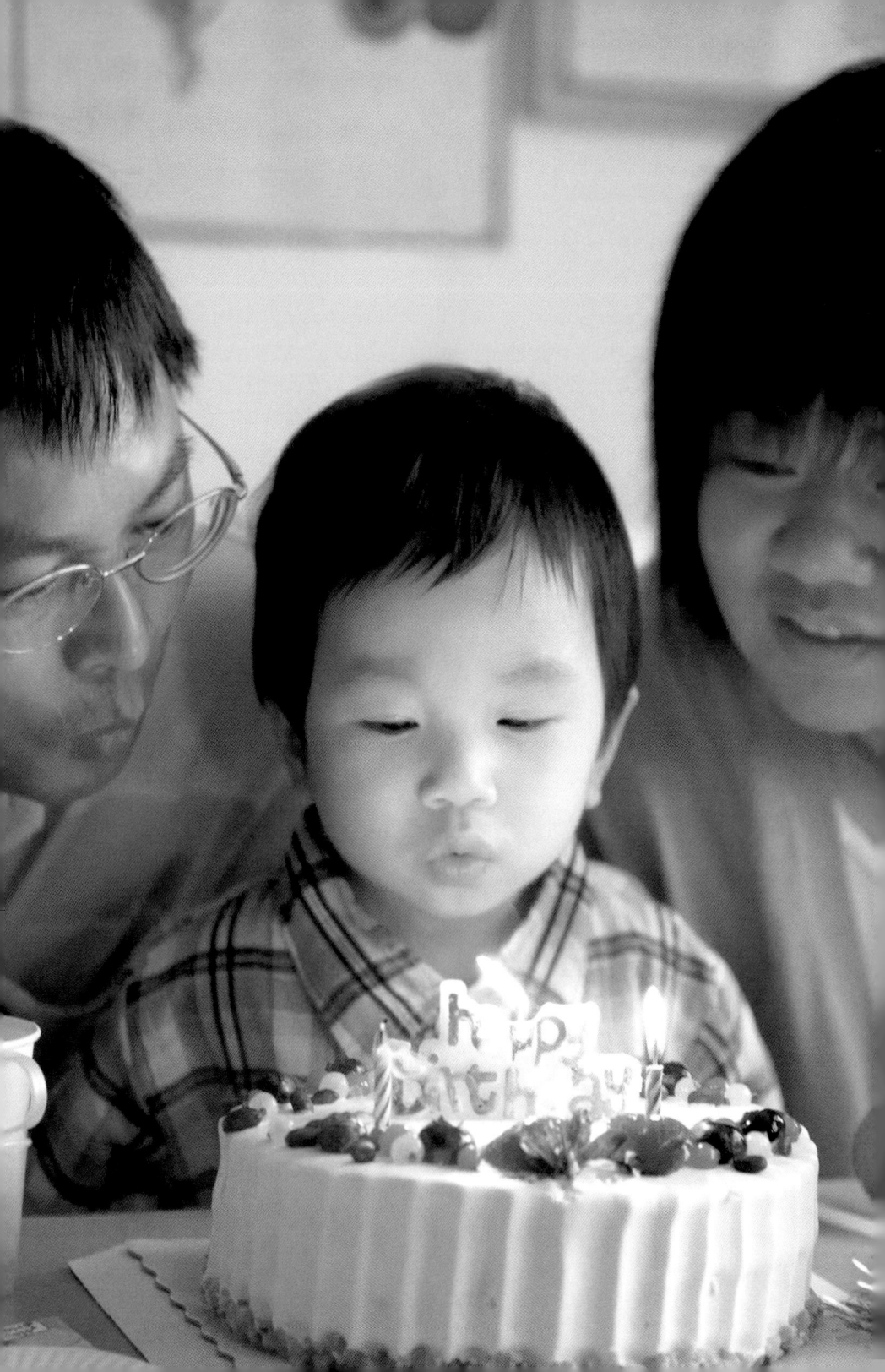

Section 2
Precious beyond words

◀ Little patient Sam and his family (see page 76 "Sam's mother")

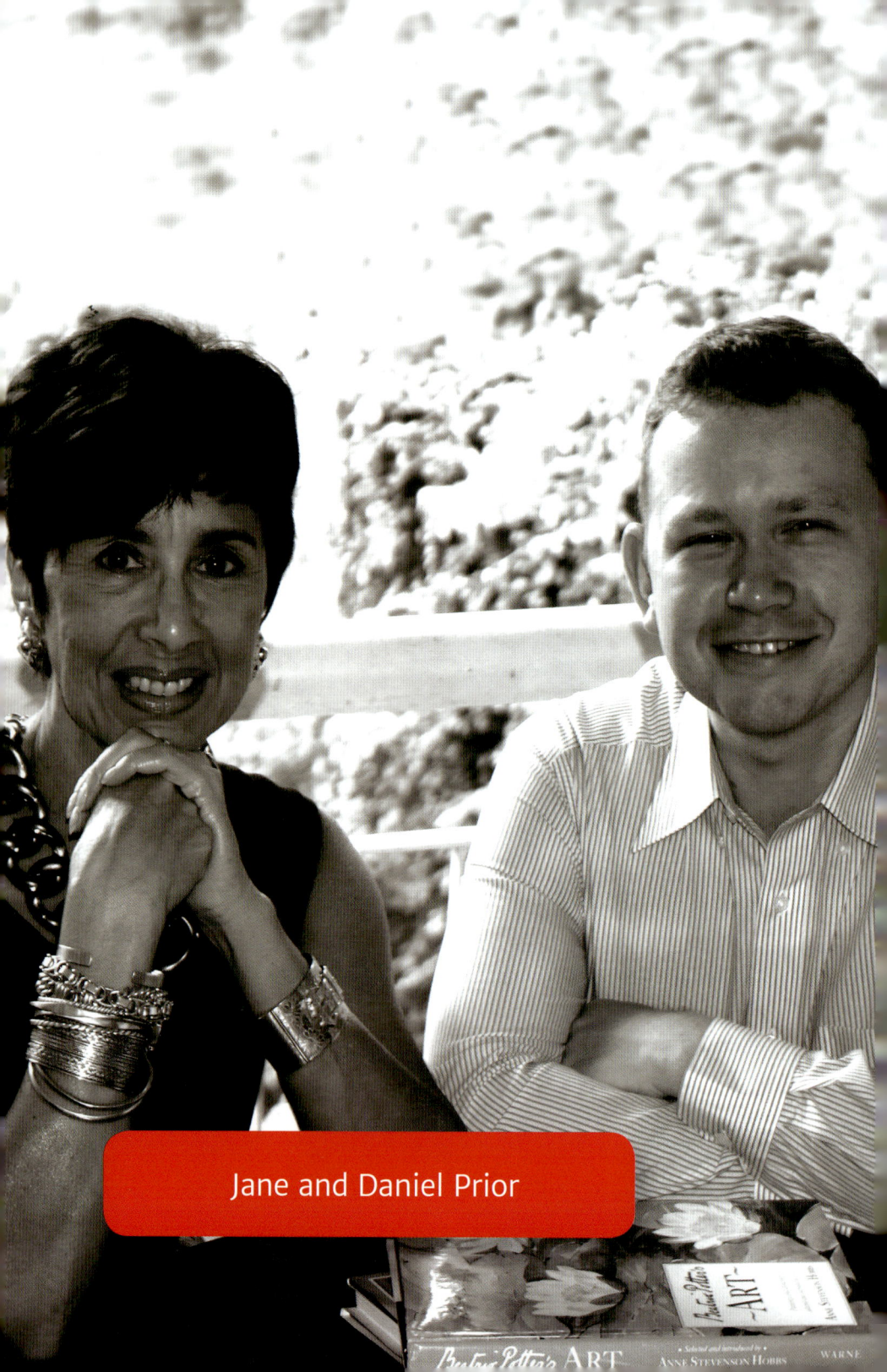

Jane and Daniel Prior

"No big deal"

*Jane Prior, mother of patient Daniel Prior
and Chief Executive of Bone Marrow Programme Singapore*

It was 1996 and our eldest son had been ill for the longest time. When he was finally diagnosed with acute myeloid leukaemia (AML), it was almost a relief to put a name to the relentless adversary that had disrupted too many childhood adventures and disturbed even more nights with endless fevers and pain.

From the outset, we were told that his only chance for survival was a bone marrow transplant and, trying to bring optimism to the darkness, the doctor said that we were "lucky because we were Caucasians". It did not mean very much on that very first morning. However, there were no matches within the family and, at that time, the local Singapore register was still a start-up with predominantly Chinese donors—so we quickly understood that Daniel's life would depend upon a match being found in the registers of Australia, the US or the UK.

Indeed, we were lucky, and just six months from the day of his diagnosis, Daniel received a transplant from a donor in Australia. We later learned that she had been turned away as a blood donor as she was older than the recommended age limit, but that she was still able to help someone as a bone marrow donor. All that was within days of Daniel's diagnosis. And Daniel now has the distinction of

> Acute myeloid leukaemia (AML) is a cancer of the myeloid line of blood cells, characterised by the rapid growth of abnormal white blood cells that build up in the bone marrow and interfere with the production of normal blood cells. AML is the most common acute leukaemia affecting adults, and its incidence increases with age.

being Singapore's first successful paediatric bone marrow transplant patient at the National University Hospital.

With remarkably little by way of side effects or complications, Daniel picked up his life again, finished school, then went to university— and he has not looked back since. From a mother's perspective, I see Daniel's recovery as the start of a personal journey. Our family is now committed to making sure that everyone in a similar situation could have the same luck.

Singapore's register, the Bone Marrow Donor Programme, recently celebrated 21 years of saving lives. We have 50,000 donors on the local register and have made the commitment to double this in the next three to five years. The challenge we face is that, while Singapore's population is fewer than six million people, it is made up of many different ethnic groups: the Chinese, Malays, Indians and a scattering of others, still arriving from every race and continent in the world. Interracial marriages are becoming more common,

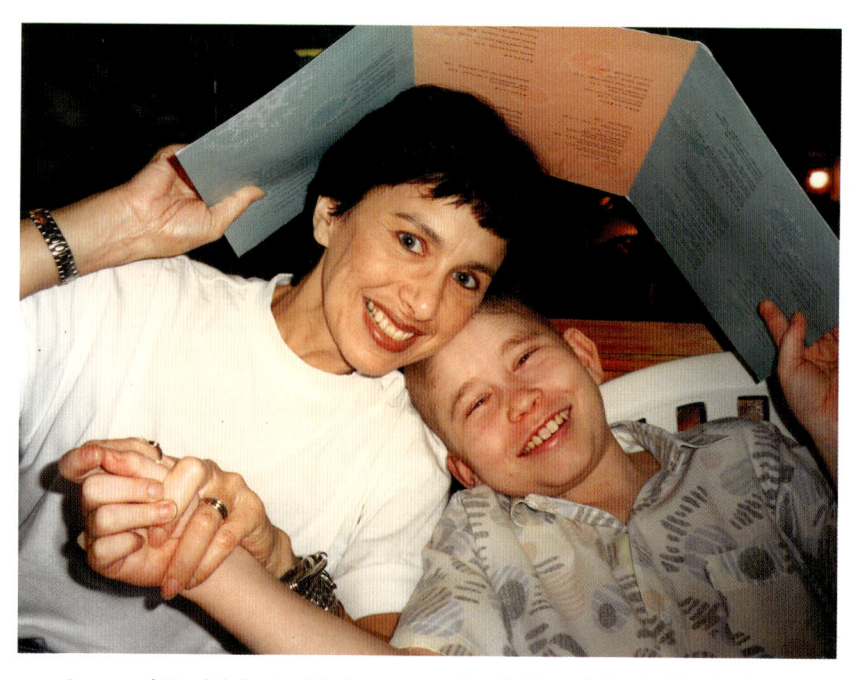

Jane and Daniel during his treatment; Daniel hasn't looked back since.

and now the children of these families are themselves looking to get married, which adds to the diversity and complexity of our population.

> "But we do win! Every day there are small victories as more donors are willing to step forward for verification typing when we tell them they have come up as a potential match."

When trying to find a matching donor for our patients, racial diversity is just one challenge. Another issue we face is that many older Singaporeans still grapple with irrational fears and age-old superstitions all compounded by a closed concept of family and commitment. Some still believe that people fall ill because they have done something wrong in a past life and that their illness is some form of retribution. This results in many patients being reluctant to be identified for the shame that it may bring on them, which makes it difficult to put a face to the diseases we are working to cure. While we can educate and instil a sense of altruism in our young people, reaching the hearts and minds of their elders is still an uphill battle.

But we do win! Every day there are small victories as more donors are willing to step forward for verification typing when we tell them they have come up as a potential match. When we ask our donors about their donation experiences, almost all of them say that it was "no big deal"; if we do our part correctly, each donor is physically fit, mentally prepared and it takes just a handful of hours for them to make that life-saving donation. Indeed, it is no big deal for the donor—but for Daniel and all the other patients who have benefited from their donations, it is the biggest deal in the world… and every day I am humbled to be a part of that.

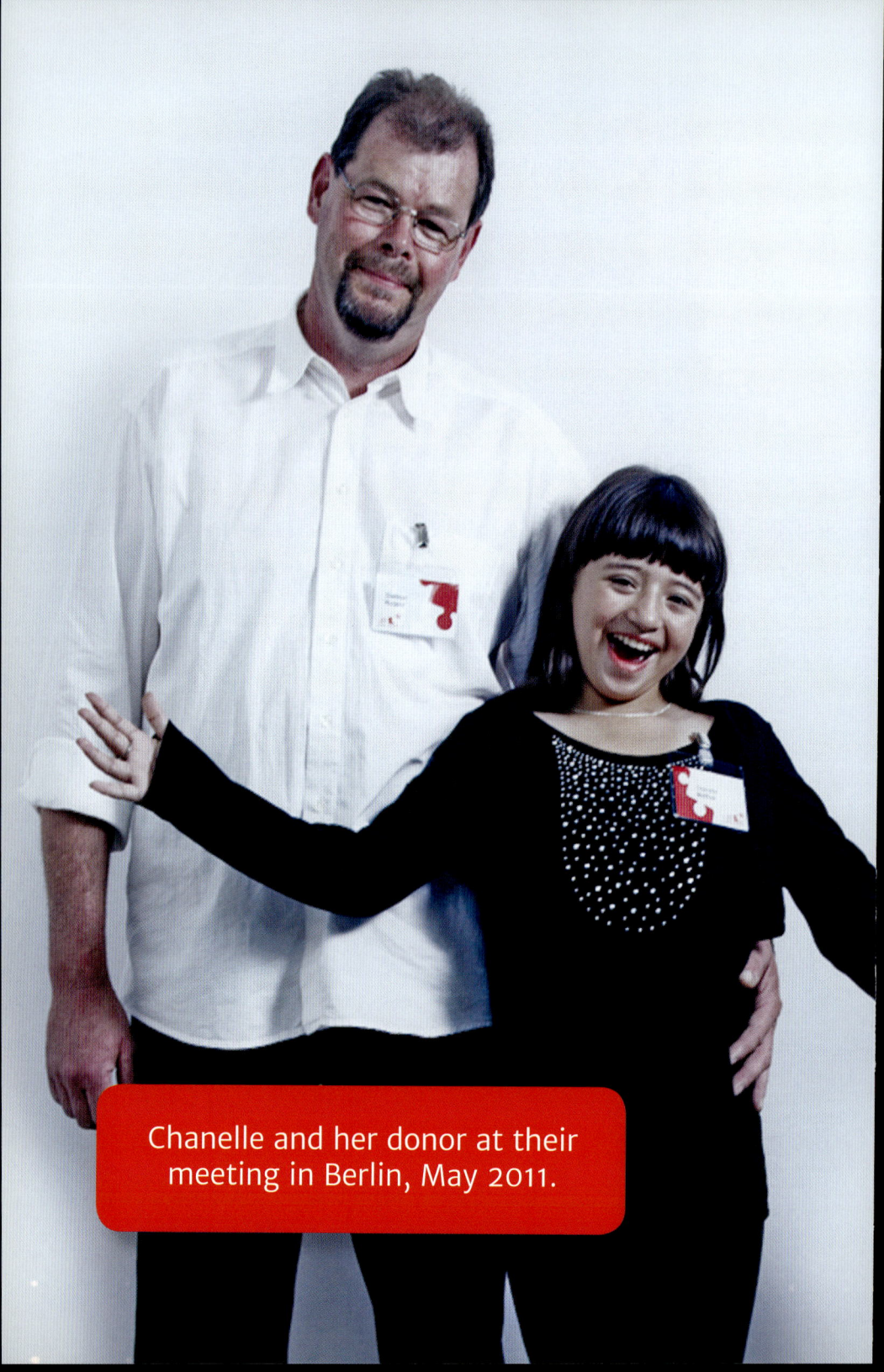

Chanelle and her donor at their meeting in Berlin, May 2011.

Courage and commitment

*Chanelle Matthee, South Africa,
recipient of bone marrow transplant in 2005*

*Written with the support of Terry Schlaphoff,
South African Bone Marrow Registry*

I was diagnosed with aplastic anaemia in 2004 when I was just five years old. By the following year, my only hope of survival was a stem cell transplant. I was referred to the South African Bone Marrow Registry (SABMR) in the hope that they could find me a suitable donor in the global database of stem cell donors.

SABMR eventually found a match for me in Germany. While the infusion went well, the stem cells that I received did not grow. The doctors waited more than three weeks and did several tests before telling me that, unfortunately, there had been no engraftment.

As I was so young at the time, I did not realise how serious my situation was. If the donor cells could not help me produce red and white blood cells and platelets, I would surely die. SABMR went back

> Aplastic anaemia is a condition that occurs when the body stops producing enough new blood cells. Aplastic anaemia leaves you feeling fatigued and with a higher risk of infections and uncontrolled bleeding. It is a rare and serious condition; aplastic anaemia can develop at any age. Aplastic anaemia may occur suddenly, or it can occur slowly and get worse over time. Treatment may include medications, blood transfusions or a stem cell transplant.

to their colleagues in Germany and asked my donor if he would be prepared to help me again—but this time by donating his bone marrow instead of peripheral blood stem cells.

> "Although the operation is generally safe and thousands of people have donated bone marrow around the world, some people hesitate out of fear. My donor showed amazing courage and commitment by agreeing to donate his bone marrow."

I now know that bone marrow donation is usually done under general anaesthesia and that the donor had to have about a litre of blood and marrow cells extracted from his pelvic bones. Although the operation is generally safe and thousands of people have donated bone marrow around the world, some people hesitate out of fear. My donor showed amazing courage and commitment by agreeing to donate his bone marrow.

And this time the transplant worked. The new cells from the donor engrafted and I am now more than five years post-transplant. In 2011, I was invited to meet my donor in Germany. It was my first trip overseas, and the first for my parents as well. We all felt a mixture of nervousness and excitement about the trip.

Finally, the big day arrived. When I met my donor for the first time, I remember how he just stopped when he saw me. I could see that he was holding back tears. It turned out that I was almost the same age as his daughter! I can only imagine how he must have felt to save the life of someone who was just as old as his own child. Since our meeting, our families have stayed in close contact and I am certain we will continue to be in touch for many years to come.

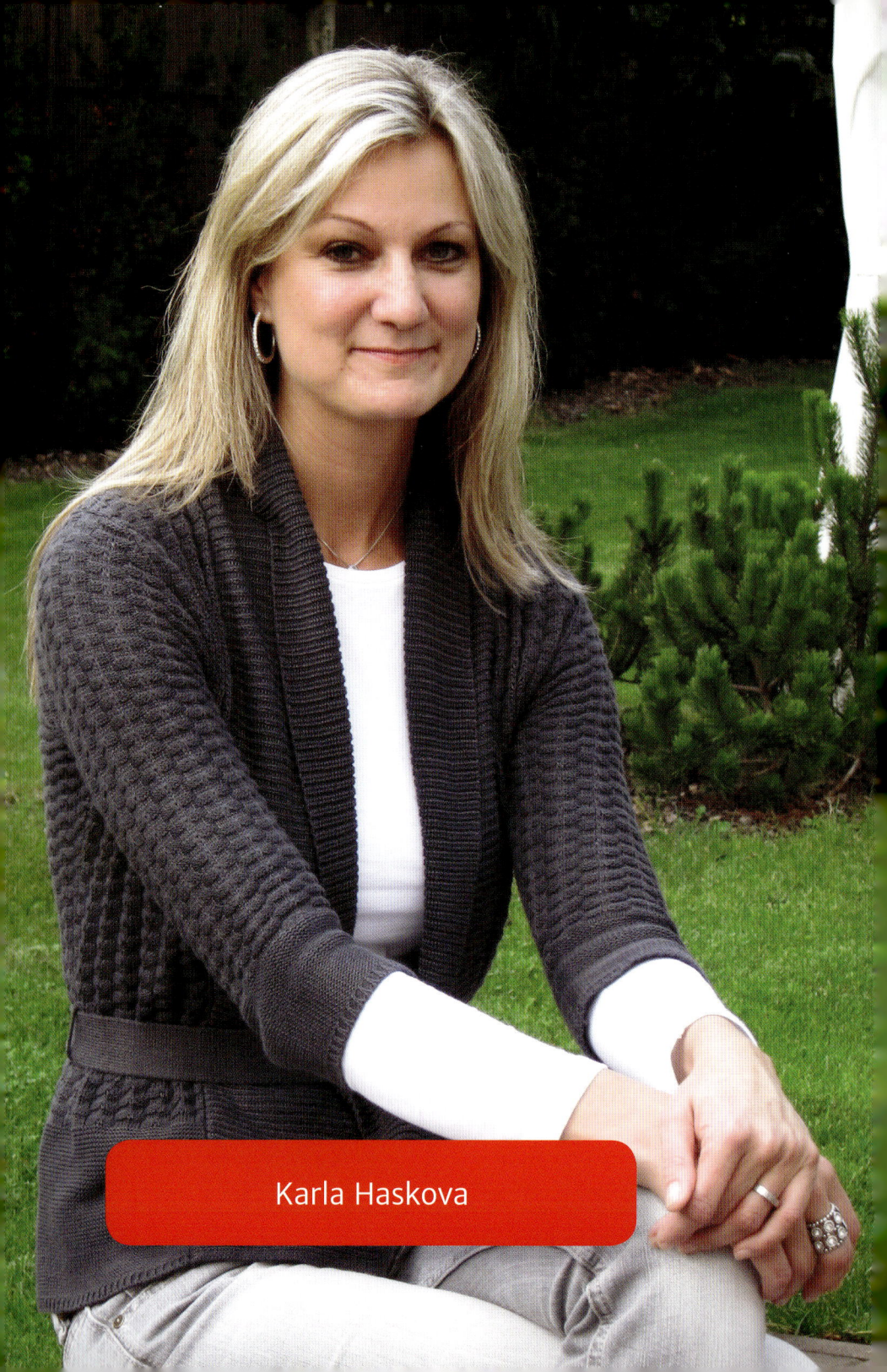

Karla Haskova

Let's proceed

*Karla Haskova, Czech Republic,
recipient of a bone marrow transplant in March 2006*

*Written with the support of Pavel Jindra,
Czech National Marrow Donors Registry*

"Karla, I really think we should go ahead with the stem cell transplant. Are you happy to proceed?" the doctor asked, looking at me for a response.

I had been asked the same question multiple times since I was diagnosed with a rare, life-threatening blood disorder called paroxysmal nocturnal haemoglobinuria in 1996. Before that, I had been a happy, sociable person and was pursuing a career as a model. But my illness had left me feeling scared. I was afraid of what the future might bring.

> Paroxysmal nocturnal haemoglobinuria (PNH) is a disorder that causes blood cells to have an increased tendency to undergo lysis (breakdown) in the blood stream. While there are drugs available to treat the disorder, the only cure is a bone marrow transplant. Some patients with PNH may develop severe aplastic anaemia, a condition in which the bone marrow stops producing adequate numbers of blood cells like red blood cells, white blood cells and platelets. A bone marrow transplant can be life-saving for sufferers of this disorder, and when a matched sibling cannot be found, an unrelated donor from one of the bone marrow registries around the world can also be used. Currently, nearly 50 per cent of patients receive stem cells from a donor who lives in another country.

After 10 years of treatment at the University Hospital in Pilsen, Czech Republic, I had developed severe aplastic anaemia and was increasingly dependent on regular blood transfusions. I knew I had to have the transplant; it could not wait any longer.

"Karla, would you like to proceed?" the doctor asked again. This time I nodded. "Yes, let's proceed."

Once I agreed to the procedure, the wheels were set in motion. A donor was found in the global database of potential stem cell donors and I went through all the necessary health checks. But on the day that operation was scheduled to take place, I was told that the potential donor they had found was unable to donate. My heart sank. A search for an alternative donor began immediately. After a few weeks, one was finally found in the US. The transplant was really happening this time—and I am so grateful that everything went according to plan.

Today I am 100 per cent healthy and finally able to realise my dreams. After the transplant, I married my long-term boyfriend, Zdenek. I also started volunteering for The Bone Marrow Transplant Foundation, which aims to improve the quality of life of others undergoing stem cell transplants in the Czech Republic.

But there is one dream I have yet to fulfil—and that is to meet the person who gave me this new chance at life.

To my saviours

An open letter from a cord blood transplant recipient to his donor

To my saviours,

Alas I will never know your address nor name because it's forbidden... but you exist somewhere, a mother and a child, not knowing where and in which country so I write in international English.

I got Leukemia, 56 years old and I'm a man... worldwide no matching donor could be found... so the doctors tried my own modificated stemcells but I relapsed and was told I only had 3 months to live... unless a last chance... and that was your matching umbilical blood they found. And up to now, after a 3 years long and heavy struggle, that saved at last my life....

I'm doing so good that my oncologist considers me as a kind of miracle but that miracle has happened in fact thanks to both of you... an unknown mother and child. How to thank you? Alas only via this poor writing.... trying to express my infinite gratitude to both of you.

May life bless both of you... you deserve it.... that's my deepest wish.

Your deeply thankful

B.

06.10.2013

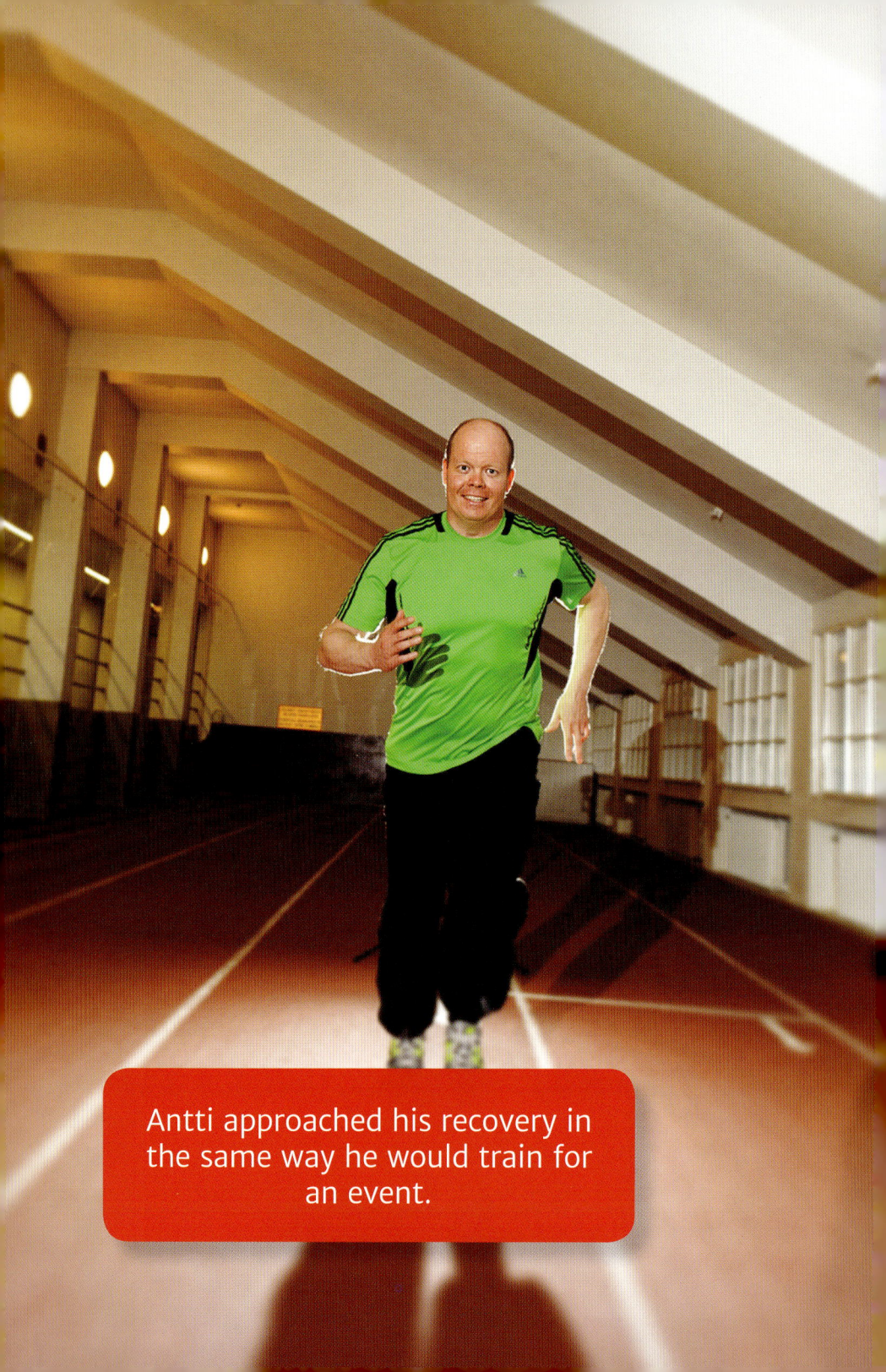

Antti approached his recovery in the same way he would train for an event.

Always moving forward

Antti Hagqvist, Finland, recipient of a stem cell transplant in December 2011

In September 2012, I lined up with thousands of others at the start of the Challenge Barcelona race. With a 3.8 km swim, 180 km bike ride and 42.2 km run ahead of me, my stomach was full of butterflies. I was not even sure I could finish the race. But then I recalled what I had experienced over the last 12 months and realised that I owed it to myself to give it my best shot.

I decided to do the race in autumn 2011, shortly after being informed that I had acute myeloid leukaemia for the second time. I had first been diagnosed 10 years earlier when I was just 24. Back then I had been treated with chemotherapy—powerful cytostatic drugs that made me sick and lose my hair, but that put the disease in remission. This time around, it was clear I would need a stem cell transplant to recover permanently.

> Chemotherapy drugs are used to kill cancer cells, which grow and divide more rapidly than normal cells. However, the drugs can also affect rapidly dividing normal cells, for example, blood cells that produce white blood cells, red blood cells and platelets, as well as hair cells and cells of normal mucous membranes (like in the mouth). That is why patients receiving chemotherapy may lose their hair, get mouth ulcers and become prone to infection.

Current chemotherapy drugs are more effective and less toxic. Many new, targeted drugs have also been developed for cancer-specific proteins. These treatments can treat and even cure many patients with blood cancers, but they are often not enough. Patients with low-risk acute myeloid leukaemia can be cured through chemotherapy, but those with high-risk AML have a very poor chance of long-term survival with chemotherapy alone. For these patients, a bone marrow transplant may represent the best chance of a long-term cure.

Patients are encouraged to do mild to moderate exercise following a transplant to help improve their cardiovascular and respiratory fitness and enhance their overall sense of well-being. In turn, these effects can lead to a better overall outcome and quality of life for the patient after transplantation. The key, of course, is to exercise in moderation and in close consultation with a physician.

Everything happened very quickly. A donor was found in Germany, and a week before Christmas I received a stem cell transplant at Turku University Hospital in Finland. On 26 December, the first white blood cells were detected in my blood samples. I could not have been happier when I was discharged from hospital on my birthday on 4 January.

The treatment I received after the transplant went unbelievably smoothly. I think it was because I approached my recovery the same way I trained for an event: I did everything I could, as well as I could. And I began exercising as soon as my doctor allowed me to—even after an infection resulted in renal

> "I approached my recovery the same way I trained for an event: I did everything I could, as well as I could."

failure and I had to rest in bed for four weeks. When I felt up to it, I would walk from one end of the corridor to the other. At first it left me so tired that I would sleep for an hour-and-a-half afterwards. But after I woke up, I was able to do the same corridor walk twice. By the time I had recovered, I was able to walk 5 km.

Four-hundred-and-thirteen days after I had received my diagnosis, I completed the Challenge Barcelona race in 12 hours and two minutes. I feel like my illness has given me a new outlook on life. I have become more comfortable in my own skin. And I have continued with my healthy lifestyle because I really believe the choices we make can help us live a long, healthy life. By always moving forward, I hope this illness will never touch me again.

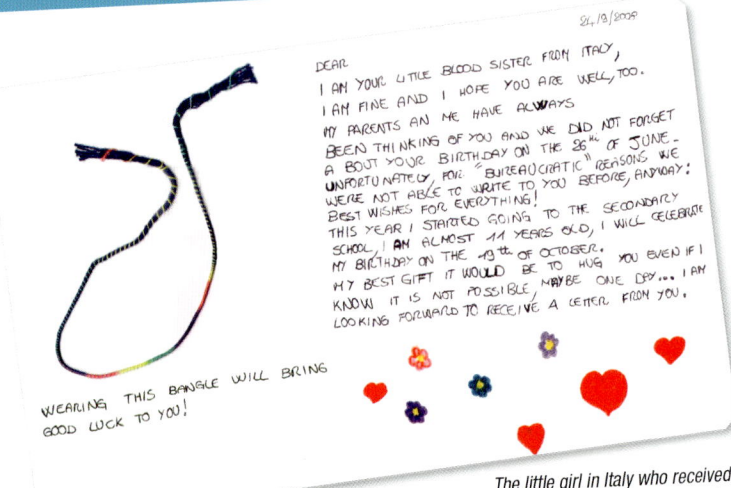

The little girl in Italy who received a life-saving transplant facilitated by the ABMDR writes to her anonymous donor

DEAR
I AM YOUR LITTLE BLOOD SISTER FROM ITALY, I AM FINE AND I HOPE YOU ARE WELL, TOO. MY PARENTS AND ME HAVE ALWAYS BEEN THINKING OF YOU AND WE DID NOT FORGET ABOUT YOUR BIRTHDAY ON THE 26TH OF JUNE. UNFORTUNATELY, FOR "BUREAUCRATIC" REASONS WE WERE NOT ABLE TO WRITE TO YOU BEFORE, ANYWAY: BEST WISHES FOR EVERYTHING!

THIS YEAR I STARTED GOING TO THE SECONDARY SCHOOL. I AM ALMOST 11 YEARS OLD, I WILL CELEBRATE MY BIRTHDAY ON THE 19TH OF OCTOBER. MY BEST GIFT IT WOULD BE TO HUG YOU EVEN IF I KNOW IT IS NOT POSSIBLE, MABYE ONE DAY . . .
I AM LOOKING FORWARD TO RECEIVE A LETTER FROM YOU.

WEARING THIS BANGLE WILL BRING GOOD LUCK TO YOU!

Birthday gifts for Boris

Patricia LaCroix, Armenian Bone Marrow Donor Registry (ABMDR)

"I wanted that unknown little girl to survive, to be able to celebrate her next birthday."
Vaheh ('Boris'), 22, Armenia, donated his stem cells in 2004

That 'little girl' has celebrated nine birthdays since her donor Vaheh (nicknamed 'Boris' by her family) made that statement in 2004. Yet she is still unknown to him, as he is to her.

They may be unknown to each other by name and sight, but not by blood or affection. Separated by 17 years and more than 1,700 miles—the girl in Italy, Boris in Armenia—they have celebrated each other's birthdays, sending each other letters, drawings and small gifts, since that miraculous match.

What Boris has done for that little girl is an affirmation of the best qualities of the human spirit. Having given her the ultimate birthday gift—the gift of life—he now receives birthday gifts every year from the grateful little girl, who now wishes him "all the joy you can have in the world". He certainly has given that to her.

These are some of the letters that the patient and her family sent to Boris to express their gratitude.

Dear boy,
In the beginning you were a hope, a distant dream. Today you are a wonderful reality. Thank you—we will keep you in our hearts forever.

A dad, a mum and a little girl

---◆---

Dear angel,
By now you are like a member of the family to us. We have given you the nickname 'Boris' and we always wonder about what you might be doing. Whether you are studying or working or going out with your friends, we always pray for your health and happiness.

We will always be thankful for the wonderful thing you did for your little Italian sister.

Your Italian mother, father and little sister

---◆---

Dear Boris,
My parents and I have been thinking of you and we did not forget about your birthday on 26 June. We hope that wearing this bangle will bring you good luck! This year I will be 11 years old and I will celebrate my birthday on 19 October. My best gift would be a hug from you, even though I know it is not possible. Maybe one day …

Your little sister in Italy

---◆---

Hi Boris,
Thanks a lot for the gifts you sent—your drawing is now beside your sister's bed. We send best wishes for your next birthday. We will raise a toast to you and hope that one day we might be possible to celebrate it together with you!

Big hug, write soon.

P.S. We are sending you a souvenir from your sister's first communion and a little present for you as well.

Dear Boris,
You do not know how happy I feel reading your letters. Thank you for the beautiful gifts. I have never asked about your life or whether you have brothers or sisters, or if you live with your parents or have a family of our own? I have two sisters, both older than I am. One is the same age as you. As 26 June is approaching and that's your birthday, I wanted to send you a bracelet with my initial on it, 'S'. I am looking forward to hearing from you and wish you all the joy you can have in the world.

S and family

Dear Angel,

We will always be thakful for the wonderful and full of love thing you did to you little italian sister.
By now, you are as a member of our family for us – we also gave you the name "Boris"- and it happens we think about what you are doing, whether you are studying or working or going out with your friends and we always pray for your health and happiness.
We hope that maybe one day we could meet, it would be a joy to put two brothers together.
Your little Italian sister is going to primary school, she is a clever and brilliant pupil, in health and we hope we can always give you good news.
We are looking forward to hearing from you and we wish you all happiness.

Your Italian mother, father and little sister

P.S. A little present for your next Birthday!

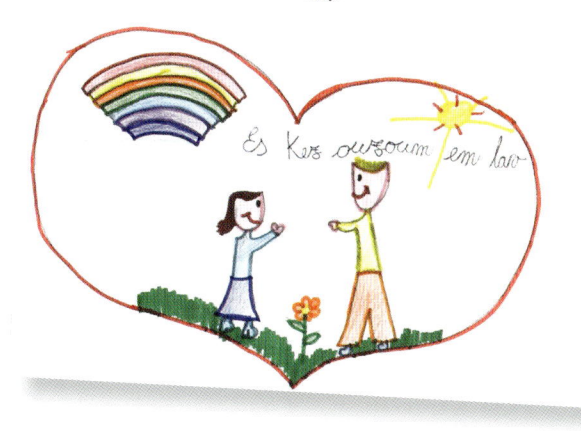

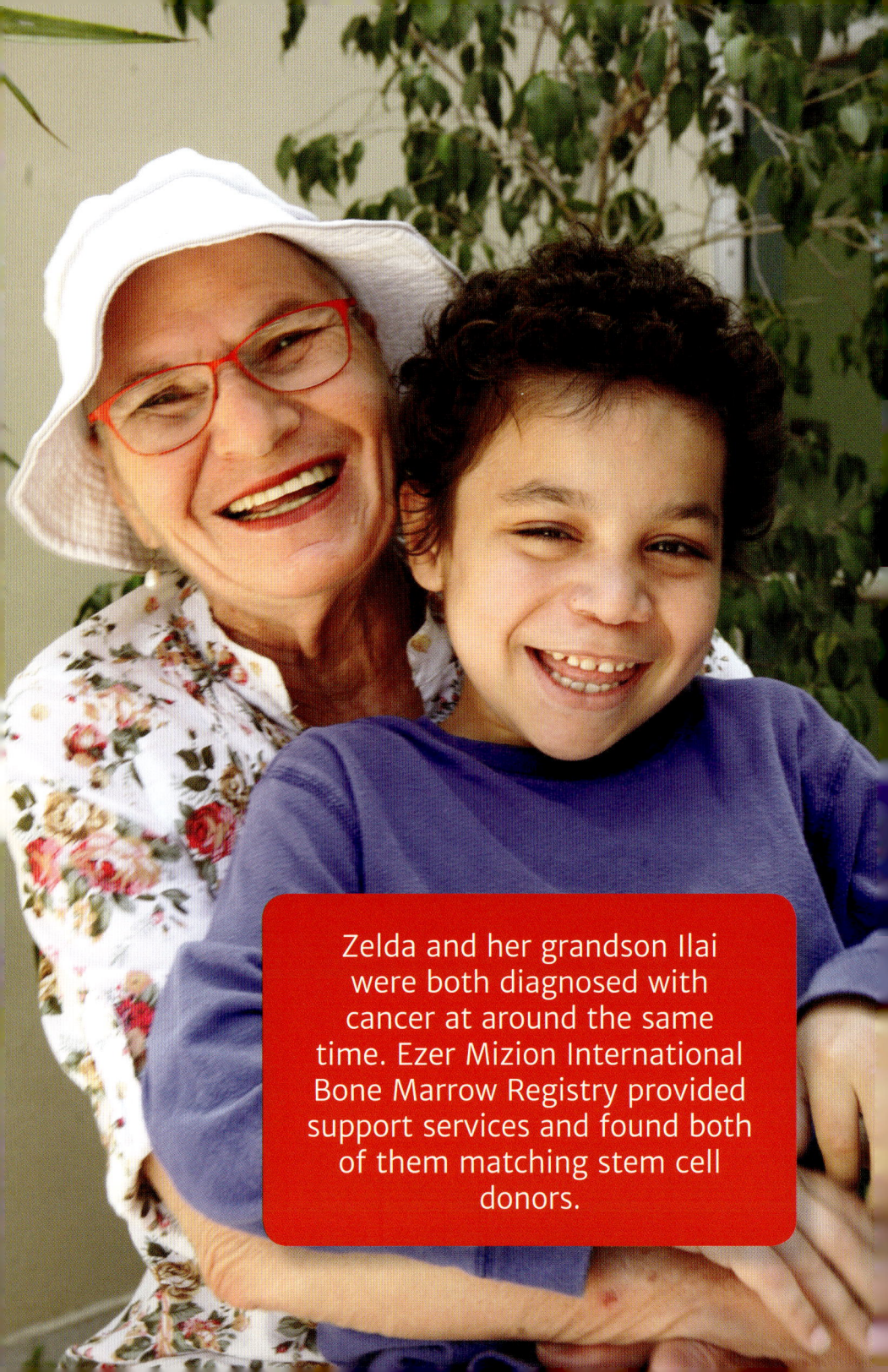

Zelda and her grandson Ilai were both diagnosed with cancer at around the same time. Ezer Mizion International Bone Marrow Registry provided support services and found both of them matching stem cell donors.

Fighting a battle on two fronts

Miki, a mother and daughter

*Written with the support of Nira Shriki,
Ezer Mizion International Bone Marrow Registry, Israel*

I was drained emotionally and physically. My six-year-old son Ilai had been battling cancer, but his chemotherapy was not working. I thought I had used up every last bit of energy and cried every last tear. And then the unthinkable happened: my 71-year-old mother, Zelda, was also diagnosed with cancer.

I watched as Ilai and his grandma Zelda rallied together to give each other strength. They were both told that a stem cell transplant was their only chance for survival. We waited, hoped and prayed while the Ezer Mizion International Bone Marrow Registry began a search for matching donors.

During that time, I became very familiar with Ezer Mizion's extensive cancer patient support services. As well as providing practical help, the organisation proved to be an invaluable source of empowerment and emotional support for our family. They brought us strength and courage.

What happened next was almost unbelievable. First, Ezer Mizion identified a match for Ilai. And just three months later, a fully compatible donor was found for his grandmother as well.

That year was tough on all of us. I shed tears until I was sure I had no tears left. But if I could choose for this not to have happened, I am not sure I would. We got to know some very special

> "It was only with the help of the wonderful staff and volunteers at Ezer Mizion that we were able to survive this ordeal, both physically and emotionally."

people at Ezer Mizion. They were with us every step of our journey and kept us going. It was only with the help of the wonderful staff and volunteers at Ezer Mizion that we were able to survive this ordeal, both physically and emotionally. These are things you only discover when you are thrust into such painful and difficult situations.

Both Ilai and Zelda recently had the good fortune to come face-to-

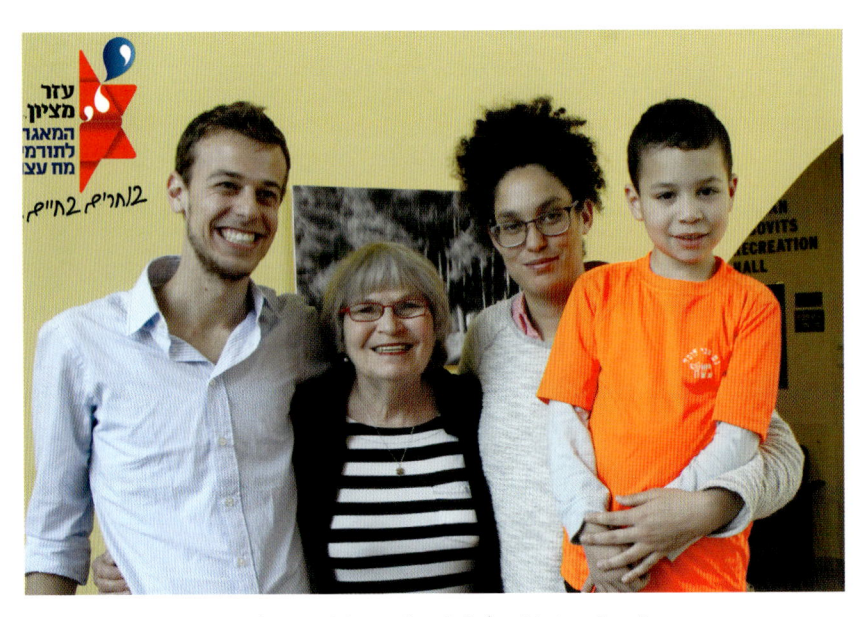

Miki (second from the right) with her family.

face with their donors. That was when I discovered that I still had tears left to shed—but this time, they were tears of gratitude and joy.

> Currently, to protect donors against coercion, unrelated donors and their recipients are not allowed to have any direct contact until a year or two after the transplant. The donation must remain a strictly altruistic and voluntary affair. When given the opportunity, patients are often keen to meet the donor whose gift saved their lives, and whose stem cells continue to live inside them, producing healthy blood cells every day. For the donors, the meeting is often an incredibly emotional experience. The practice of allowing donors and patients to meet varies between countries, as the laws and customs of different parts of the world have to be respected.

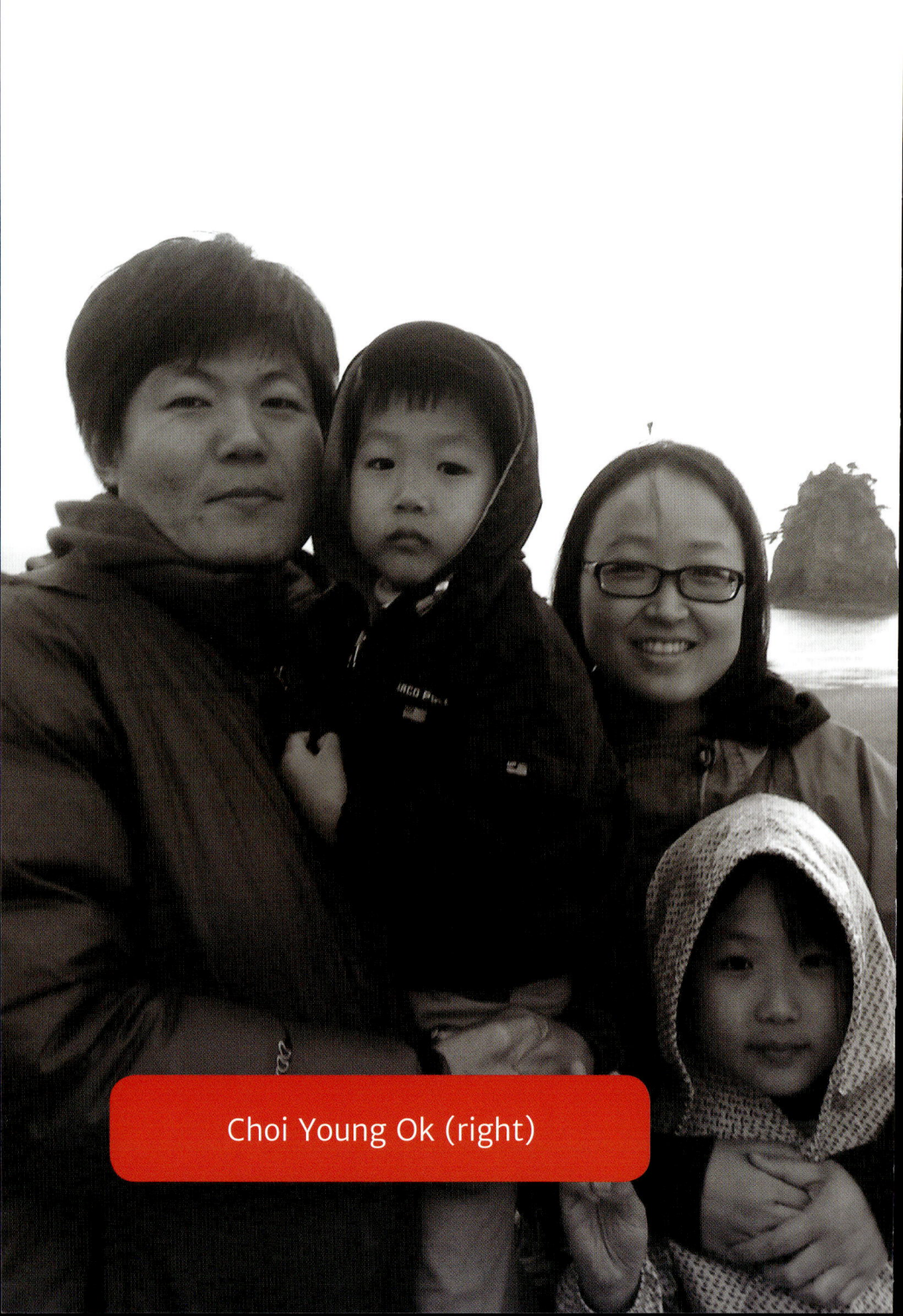

Choi Young Ok (right)

Search for meaning

Choi Young Ok, South Korea, received a transplant in 2010

It was a cold day in January when I experienced the heaviest snowfall of my life. That day, I had to wrestle my way to the hospital to deliver my second child—but that day also became a turning point in my life for another reason.

Apart from the severe anaemia that I had suffered from during my pregnancy, I was otherwise healthy. However, after my delivery, blood tests showed that my red blood cell count was just 4.0, and because I also had abnormal blood cells I was told it could be leukaemia. I underwent a bone marrow test at the hospital and was diagnosed with myelodysplastic syndrome.

My husband and I were in shock and wondered whether we could even dare to hope that I could ever recover. As a high-risk patient, I was quickly put on a course of chemotherapy and prepared for a stem cell transplant. I vowed to myself that I would fight my disease. But because I had to have surgery for all kinds of infections, I was unable to take care of myself, let alone my two-month-old baby. I had to send my oldest child to stay with my in-laws and my second child to my parents.

> Myelodysplastic syndromes (MDS) are a group of disorders caused by poorly formed or dysfunctional blood cells. Myelodysplastic syndromes occur when something goes wrong in the bone marrow (the spongy material inside our bones where blood cells are made). The number and quality of blood-forming cells decline irreversibly, further impairing blood production.

Looking back, I think that this difficult period helped me to cope with my transplant, which proved even more difficult than the chemotherapy. The worse my pain was, the more I summoned my inner strength, as if I were climbing a mountain. I forced myself to find an emotional and spiritual rock to cling to as I struggled with the pain.

> "I forced myself to find an emotional and spiritual rock to cling to as I struggled with the pain."

Whenever I felt anxious about what lay ahead, I kept repeating a quote from Nietzsche to myself, which I had read in Viktor Frankl's *Man's Search for Meaning*: "Those who have a 'why' to live, can bear with almost any 'how'."

The book says that life is like a blank sheet of paper. It is up to you to fill that empty space. So the question is not, "Why do I have to suffer this pain?" but, "How should I cope with this situation?" In other words, my life is not dictated by my circumstances, but by how I think and feel.

By considering this period of time as a 'sabbatical' during which I could rest and recover, so that I could lead a healthy and happy life with my wonderful family, I found consolation and reflection. It gave me a reason to fight my disease. It gave me a sense of duty because I was not only living my life for myself, but for others as well. I had often wondered why cancer patients often say that they are grateful for their experience, but now I have come to understand these words. When I used to say 'thank you', I did not really understand what being truly thankful meant ... But now I understand why life and its people are so precious.

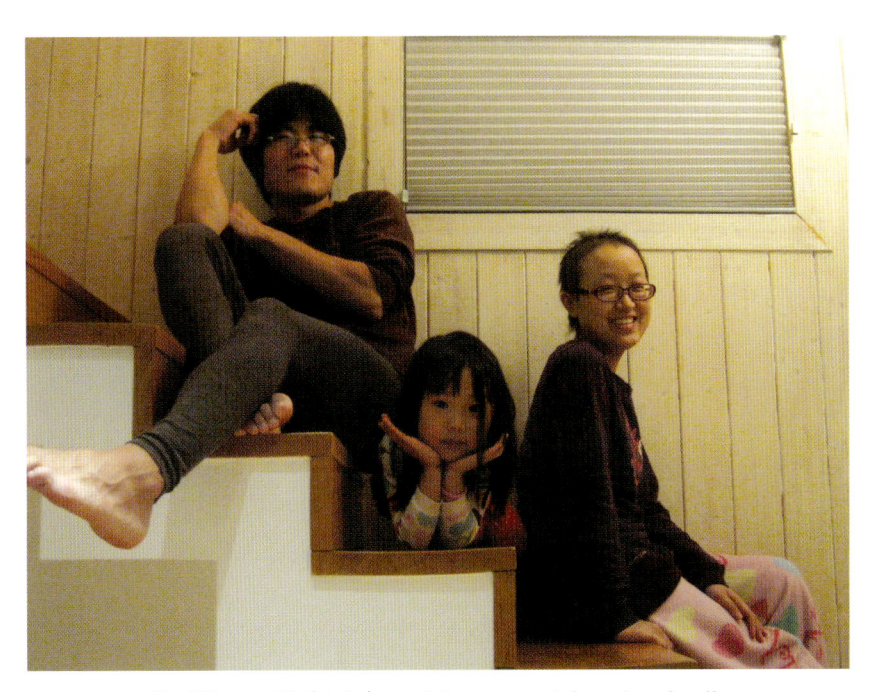

Choi Young Ok (right) receiving support from her family

In the early days of our marriage, I used to complain a lot to my husband. But since being released from the hospital, I am just so grateful to know that he is within arm's length when we go to sleep. Just being together is true happiness and bliss. Now I understand that happiness is found in the time you spend with the people you love.

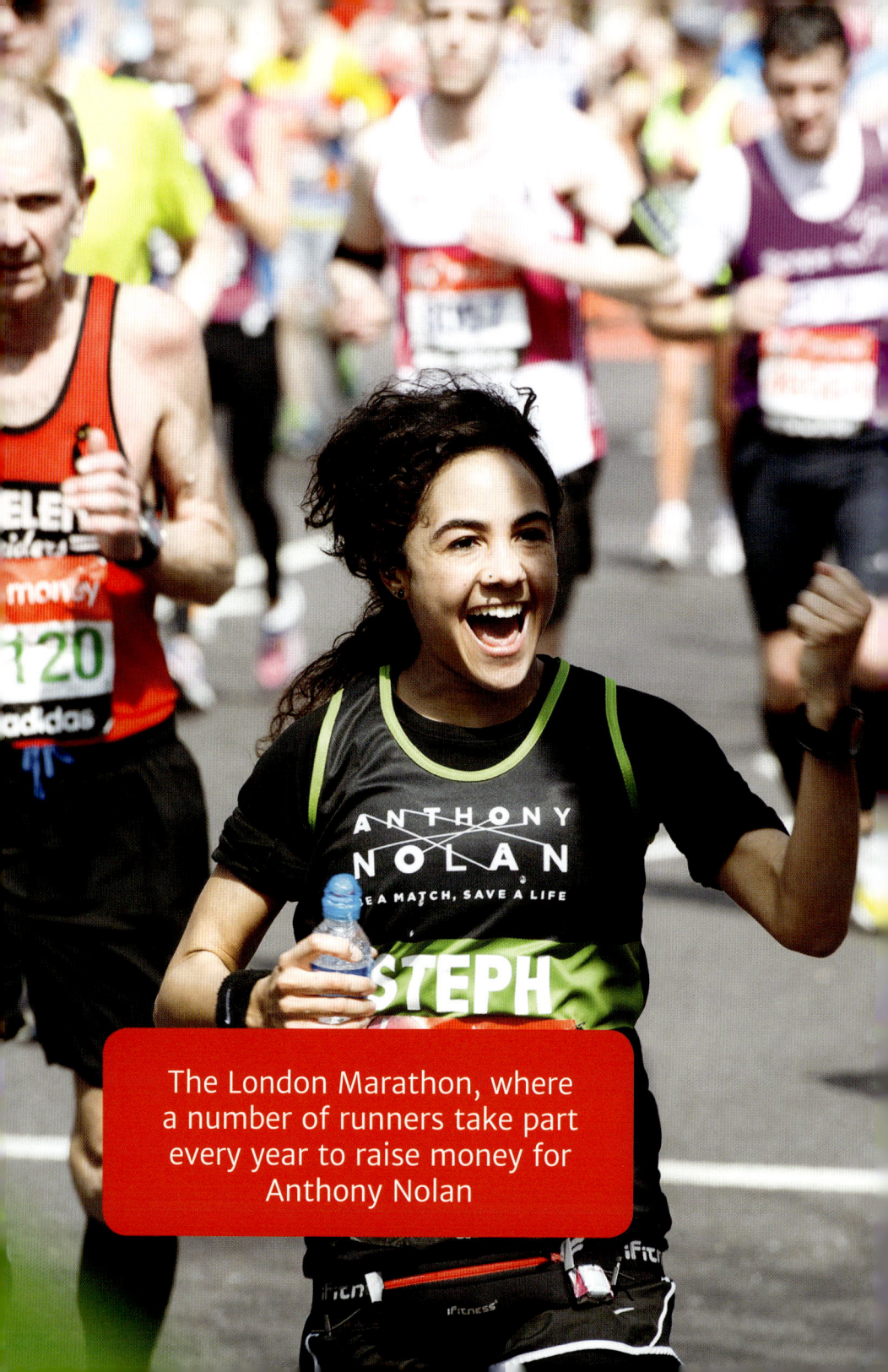

The London Marathon, where a number of runners take part every year to raise money for Anthony Nolan

New perspectives

Rizwana Rashid, recipient of an unrelated stem cell transplant in August 2009. She joined Anthony Nolan in 2010 and was their Commercial Manager.

Written with the support of Jo Badger and Emma Radway-Bright at Anthony Nolan.

In 1995 I developed a cold that I could not get rid of, despite being treated with antibiotics. My family doctor sent me for routine blood tests that picked up that I had low neutrophils. This was the worst news I could have heard as my older sister, Shabnum, had been diagnosed with a similar condition in 1987 and had unfortunately died five years later. At the time of diagnosis I thought that I, like my sister, would only have five years left.

My entire perspective changed. I decided to get on with my life and make something of it, so I graduated and started work. I relocated to Leeds and was cared for very well at Leeds Teaching Hospital. I was admitted there whenever I developed infections and needed treatment with intravenous antibiotics, which typically happened about once a year.

By the time I moved to London and started treatment at King's College Hospital, my health had deteriorated. I felt unwell all the time and my energy levels were low. My mouth was constantly sore due to painful ulcers and my skin had developed open wounds. Looking back, I realise that my decision to move to London saved my life. King's thoroughly reviewed my situation to form a more complete diagnosis, which meant lots of blood tests, bone marrow biopsies and X-rays.

In 2008 I was diagnosed with myelodysplastic syndrome (MDS—a disease in which blood production is disorderly and ineffective), and subsequently underwent a Campath trial. This unfortunately did not help. The drug was supposed to get rid of my immune system in the hope that my bone marrow would then kick-start and produce healthy cells. The trial was successful in eradicating my immune system, but my bone marrow refused to cooperate! Instead, I developed numerous infections and had to be re-admitted to King's each time.

It was at this point that my doctor decided we should give stem cell transplantation a try. So in January 2009 the search for a donor began. Given my family history, it was decided that it would be better to look for an unrelated donor, and Anthony Nolan was contacted. I feared that no match would be found because I am from an ethnic minority and no match had been found for my sister when she was ill.

So I cannot describe my joy—and my initial disbelief—when matches were identified (yes, there were more than one!).

Later that year, I was admitted to hospital for my transplant. I was kept in an isolation unit for four weeks. (I was told it would be six, but was let out two weeks early as my bone marrow was on good behaviour!)

> "I cannot describe my joy—and my initial disbelief—when matches were identified (yes, there were more than one!)"

The transplant has improved my life to an amazing extent. I feel so much better, my fitness levels have increased tremendously and I have much more energy than before. I completed the Leeds Half

Marathon in 2014, which for me, was an incredible achievement. After the event, I wrote to my donor and told him that his kind, selfless act had allowed me to get back to living my life.

Now I really value the simple things in life. I had seen what had happened to my sister and met patients at King's who were not suitable for transplants, or who sadly died after receiving one. I realise that I am very fortunate. My hope for the future is that more patients have my experience, as opposed to my sister's. That is why I would like to plead with people reading this to contact Anthony Nolan (or your own local bone marrow registry) and join the register, especially if you are from an ethnic minority.

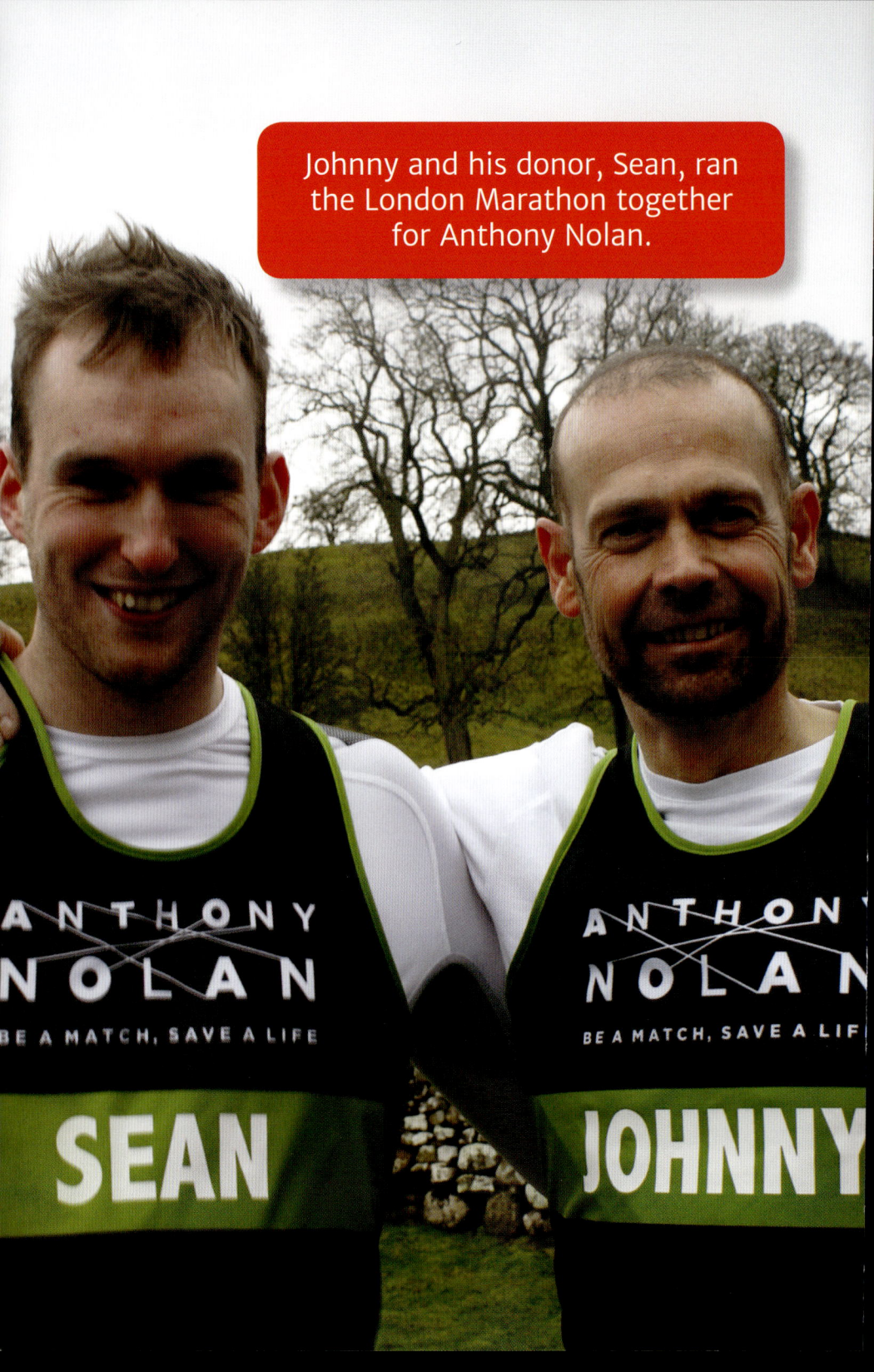

Johnny and his donor, Sean, ran the London Marathon together for Anthony Nolan.

Running mates

Johnny Pearson, UK, recipient of a bone marrow transplant in 2012

One Thursday in September, I went to see the doctor after feeling slightly under the weather and he did a blood test, "just to make sure". The next day, I was driving home from work when I got a call telling me that something was seriously wrong with the test results and that I needed to go straight to the hospital. When I was told it was leukaemia, it was the worst possible news. I thought that my life was over.

I started treatment on the following Tuesday. Six months of gruelling chemotherapy later, I was finally in remission and well enough to go home to my lovely wife, Sarah, and my boys, Jack and Archie.

But that July, just one month after returning to work, I received the devastating news that my leukaemia had relapsed. My last hope was a bone marrow transplant—and the race was on to find a matching donor.

It was a very difficult time for my family and me, as we knew that my life was in someone else's hands. Several months passed, which felt like the longest few months of my life. Then one day, my doctor sat me down and told me that Anthony Nolan had found a donor. A total stranger was willing to save my life with his bone marrow. After the transplant, I wanted to thank my donor. We were allowed to write to each other anonymously, and we soon built up a friendship. In 2013, I wrote to ask if he would like to run the London Marathon with me for Anthony Nolan the next year—and he agreed.

I had done the Great North Run before I fell ill, and at the finish line I was so exhausted that I vowed I would never do a full marathon.

But getting a second chance at life changed my mind. Running the marathon was a way for me to show how far I had come and to give something back. Without Anthony Nolan and my donor, I would not be here today; it is as simple as that.

> "I had done the Great North Run before I fell ill, and at the finish line I was so exhausted that I vowed I would never do a full marathon. But getting a second chance at life changed my mind."

In February 2014, two years after my transplant and a few months before the marathon, I was finally able to meet Sean, my donor, for the first time. It was one of the best moments of my life. How can you possibly give sufficient thanks to someone who has given you back your life?

Miracles of life

Various authors
Stories written with the support of Ruby Huang,
Marketing Director at Bionet Corp

Mr Chiou
I had always considered myself young, fit and healthy. But after a routine health check at the age of 36, I was given the devastating news that I had aplastic anaemia—a potentially fatal blood disease. Doctors told me that my only option for a cure was to undergo haematopoietic stem cell transplantation. Fortunately, the medical team identified my sister as an HLA match. Within just a few months, I made a full recovery. To this day, my sister and I can hardly believe that the cure to my disease was in her blood.

Ms Lin
I was 20 years old and had just landed my dream job in the army, so I was filled with hope for my future—until I was diagnosed with Hodgkin's lymphoma.

Unfortunately, after many months of painful chemotherapy, the disease still had not gone into remission. My doctors recommended stem cell transplantation as a last resort, but my HLA type did not match that of my sisters or other family members.

> In Hodgkin's lymphoma, cells in the lymphatic system grow abnormally and may spread beyond the lymphatic system. As the disease progresses, it compromises the body's ability to fight infection.

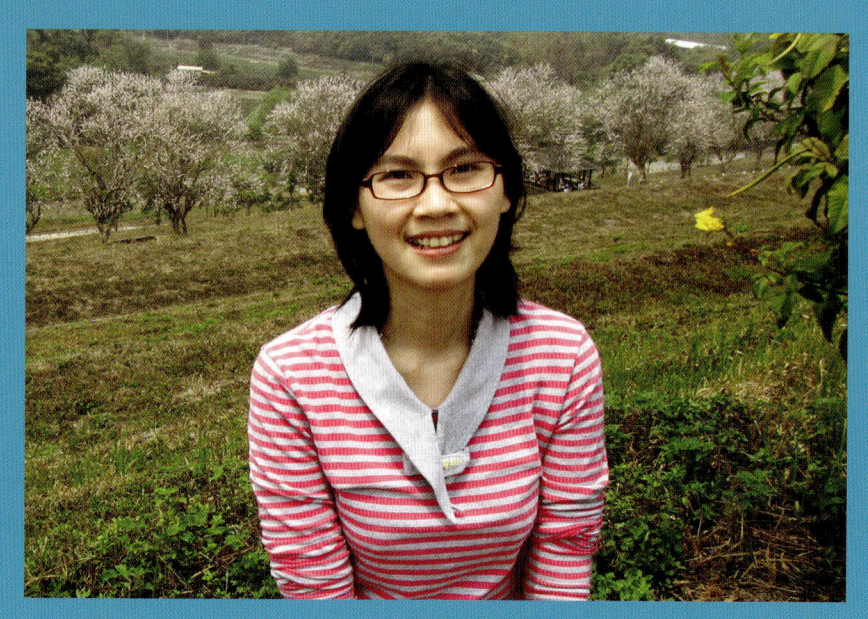

Ms Lin

Finally, a cord blood match was found. At that time, cord blood transplantation was not a common treatment option, and I was told that it could have severe consequences. But I put aside my fears and decided to go through with the procedure. The outcome proved that I made the right decision; I am now back to full health.

Sam's mother
We had previously lost two sons to a genetic disease and we were praying that our third would be free from this cruel affliction. But sadly, shortly after he was born, Sam began to experience all the same strange symptoms his brothers had. We were terrified and wondered whether this would always be our family's fate.

Fortunately, this time, the medical team was able to identify a potential cure for Sam's disease. They recommended cord blood transplantation. And thankfully, the transplant went perfectly.

Today, little Sam is able to go outside and play again—which is all thanks to the cord blood donor and the efforts of the medical team. When Sam grows up, we will tell him that he owes his health to a stranger's generosity and that it should be cherished. Hopefully, he will want to give back to society and help other people in the future.

> When a patient is unable to find a fully matched unrelated donor, a partially matched cord blood unit with an adequate cell dose may also be used. Patients receiving umbilical cord blood transplants (UCBTs) experience a slower recovery of their blood counts than those receiving marrow from an adult donor. However, compared to bone marrow transplants, UCBTs offer a lower incidence of a phenomenon known as graft-versus-host disease, where the donor's immune cells may sometimes attack the patient. As a result, the long-term outcomes of UCBTs are similar to those of fully matched marrow transplants.

Soon-ok at the orphanage in 1975

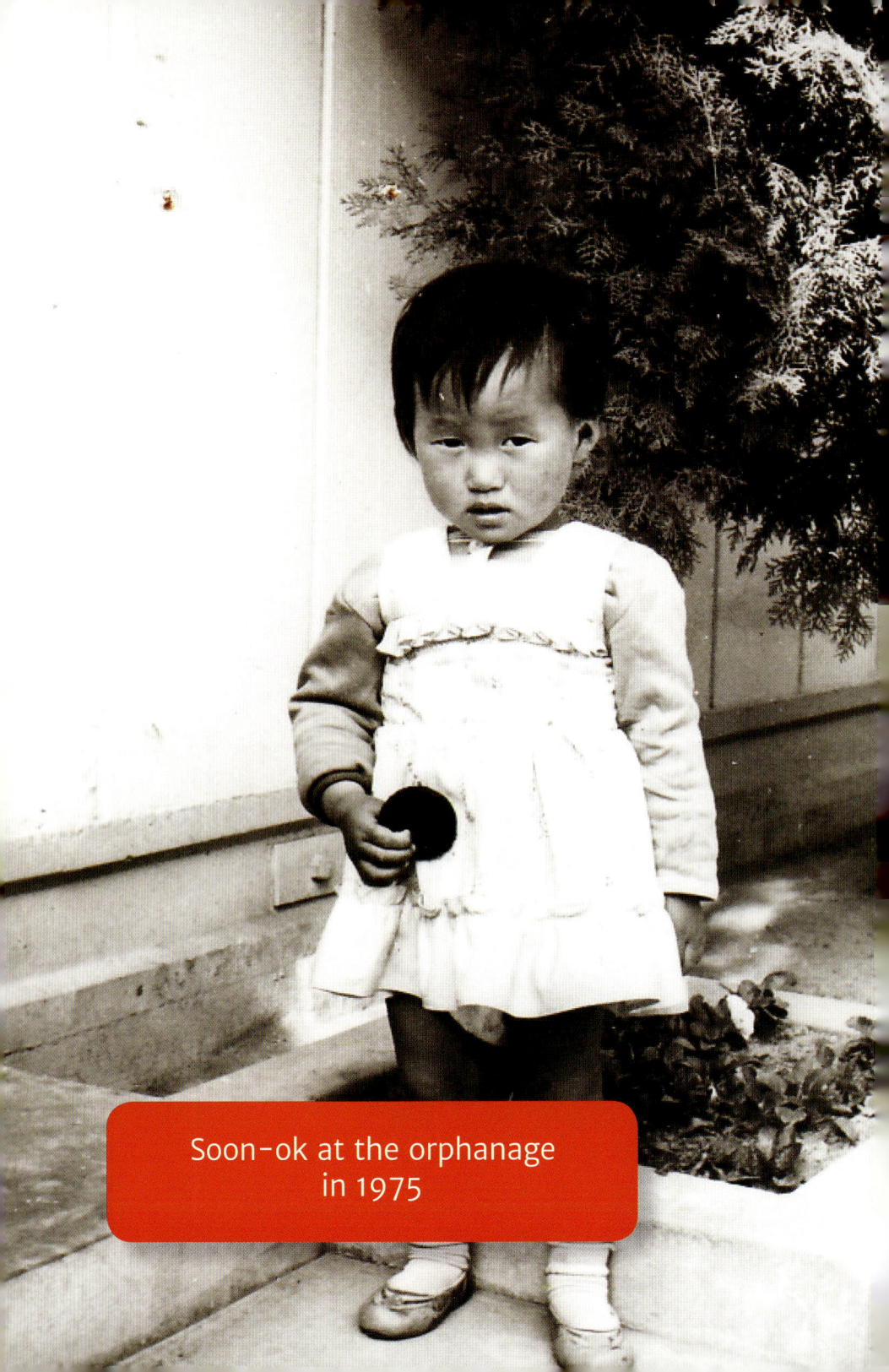

Traces of you:
A tale of love found, lost, then found again

Soon-ok Heijmans, recipient of a stem cell transplant for treatment of acute myeloid leukaemia in 2011

The story begins in Seoul, South Korea, sometime in the early 1970s, as the country awakens as an emerging economy. But in an old neighbourhood, perched high on a hill on the outskirts of Seoul, many ordinary citizens are still struggling to make ends meet. It is in one of its ramshackle houses that a hearing impaired couple have a daughter whom they eventually sent to the Netherlands to be adopted by another couple, in the hope that she will have a better future.

Twenty years later, this daughter has returned to Seoul as an exchange student. As she rides the subway on her daily commute to Yonsei University, she studies the faces of the people sitting across from her; the faces of the middle-aged men and women who had built up South Korea from the ashes of the Korean War, and that reveal a lifetime of hardship and struggle. She suddenly realises that any of these faces could well belong to her biological father or mother.

On an earlier trip to Seoul, she visited the orphanage where she had lived, only to learn that no one there knew anything about her biological parents. In a way, she felt relieved. There was no need for her to worry about the impact that the search might have on her life, or on that of her parents. But in a country that has overcome repeated foreign attacks and many hardships on the road to peace and prosperity, people take pride in the blood, sweat and tears that they share. 'I' equals 'we', and 'we' are 'one'. A taxi driver, quick to notice her faltering Korean, reminds her: "You are not Dutch. Your blood is Korean, so you are Korean."

As she wanders through the crowded streets of Seoul, experiencing life as an outsider within the skin of an insider, she is unaware that, just a few kilometres away, her Korean father, old, weak and worn down by cirrhosis of the liver, has gathered his final strength to climb up the steep hill to the orphanage where he once left her. In a last-ditch effort to see his offspring, he visits the orphanage several times, panting and sweating as he collects his breath sitting on the porch. Eager for more news, he is saddened each time when he learns that no letter has arrived yet.

A few months after their daughter had been put up for adoption, a second daughter was born and the couple had to give this child up for adoption too. Since then, the father had spent his days surviving on a small government grant. The couple's story would have remained unknown, and their significance as parents a mere footnote in the life of their daughter, had the father's cry of distress not reached her adopted parents in the Netherlands.

> "...it turns out that the younger daughter was also adopted by a Dutch family, and the two girls have grown up within an hour's drive of one another."

Sadly, the father passes away before he can be reached by the Dutch family. However, his children are eventually united. In a stroke of

United by blood, two but together

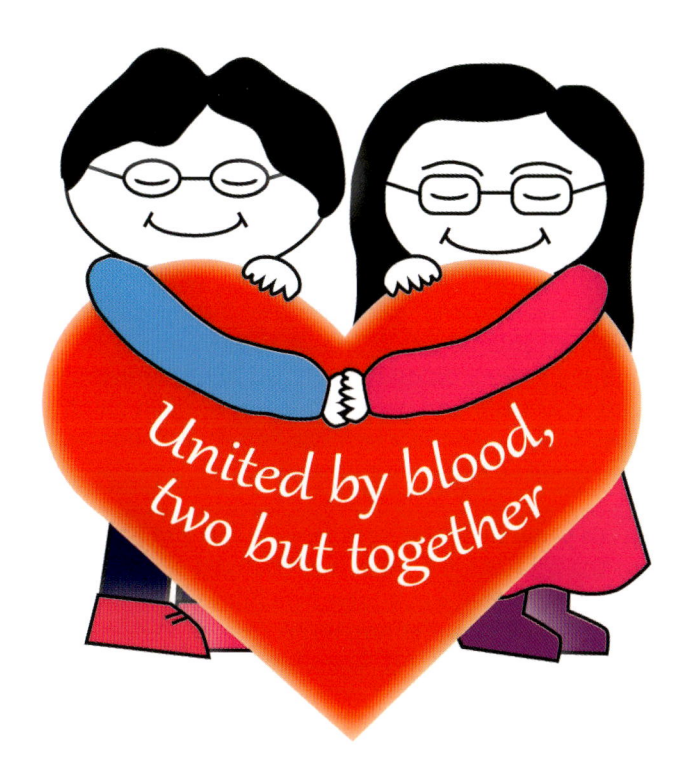

luck, it turns out that the younger daughter was also adopted by a Dutch family, and the two girls have grown up within an hour's drive of one another. In the years that follow, the sisters get to know each other, and gradually a friendship between them forms. But it's only many years later that the true meaning of their newly discovered sisterhood is revealed. And it is then that their birth father's last wish proves to be a blessing for the elder daughter.

In 2011, she is diagnosed with acute leukaemia, and only her younger sister's stem cells can save her life. Suddenly, blood ties are crucial to her very existence. She now has a 25 per cent chance of a related donor match. Amazingly, tests reveal that her younger sister is a perfect match, providing the ultimate proof that they really are sisters. Thanks to her younger sister's stem cells, she survives. At last, the taxi driver is proven right: blood is thicker than water. However, in an unsettling twist of events, the younger sister is diagnosed with an aggressive form of stomach cancer the following year. Sadly, the elder sister cannot save her—but the younger sister's blood will continue to flow in the elder sister.

This is the story of my father, my sister and I, and the bond that connects us through life and death. Our lives, which all took very different routes, were woven back together by my father's final wish and my sister's invaluable gift of life. It is through the traces they have left and my sister's blood running through my veins that I can feel the bond of kinship and protection. Never again will I be alone; I will carry my sister with me wherever I go. Her blood has become my blood, and my life has become her life.

In summer 2013, my husband, brother-in-law and I climbed up the steep hill to the orphanage. Much had changed since my first visit in 1992. It was no longer a last stop for children sent to be adopted by new families in different countries. A change in Korean law had put a halt to overseas adoption. The cheerful sounds of children running around had disappeared, leaving only the empty rooms and playground as silent witnesses of a history long gone.

Returning to the orphanage, I felt as if I had come full circle, back to the place where the lives of my father, my sister and I had taken a momentous turn. Tracing the steps our lives had taken from there and the fate that had brought us back together, I realised once more how unbelievably lucky I had been, and how precious the gift was that my father and sister had given me.

It is now summer 2014, and there has been another change of scenery. My Indian husband and I have moved back to India, where I had first been diagnosed with leukaemia. Like so many other Indian families at this time of year, we are celebrating 'Raksha Bandhan'. To mark this auspicious day, millions of sisters tie a 'rakhi' (a sacred bracelet made of interwoven threads) around the wrists of their brothers. With this ritual they bless their brothers, while reminding them of their duty to protect their sisters. The 'rakhi' is the symbol of sibling love and protection, and reaches beyond immediate family ties. On 'Raksha Bandhan', every Indian boy and man wears his "rakhi" with pride.

On this day, I imagine symbolically tying 'rakhis' around the wrists of my sister and father, family and friends, as well as the doctors and nurses of the haematology ward at Leiden University Medical Centre, where I was treated.

In a world that is filled with conflict and violence, I find it a comforting thought that anonymous donors are willing to give their stem cells to save the lives of patients they do not know, sometimes on the other side of the world. Maybe the German philosopher, Friedrich von Schiller, was right after all, and all people will become brothers and sisters eventually.

This story is dedicated to my Korean father, who truly came to life for me after his death, and to my dear sister, who will always remain a part of me.

> "Everything in the universe leaves an indelible mark—or a subtle trace—on everything it encounters. We are all a product of each other."
> Anoushka Shankar, sitar player/composer

An open letter

Sent by the recipient of a transplant in 2010 to his donor

Dear donor,
I am the young man who has a second chance at life thanks to you. Though a year has already passed since I received your stem cells, it is only now that I am sending you my gratitude for the pain you went through. I would have liked to visit you and thank you in person, but since this is not allowed, I hope you will not feel disappointed that I am sending you my gratitude this way.

After the usual heavy rains of summer, autumn has suddenly arrived on our doorstep, and I am wondering how you are doing. Though the days are hot and sultry, the mornings and evenings have become pretty chilly, so please take good care of your health.

I have recovered quite well from the transplant. But after the long fight with my disease, I still have to be very careful and there are all kinds of restrictions on the things I am allowed to do. I am studying hard to make my dreams come true, and I envy my friends who have had more time to create happy memories for themselves. But when I look back at my life, I am very grateful for everything I have.

My journey began shortly after joining the military. I found the drills so tough that I wasn't sure if my body could withstand them. I had hardly ever been ill, and even when I was sick previously I always tried to endure it, so I tried to cope. But this time the symptoms were so severe that I had to get a check-up. So, the day before our marching drill, I had a blood test and discovered that there was something wrong with my body. I was diagnosed with leukaemia, an illness that I'd only heard about on television and in movies.

While I was confined to the hospital and undergoing awful chemotherapy, I was often resentful, asking myself, "Why did this happen to me?" I cried a lot in frustration after my first autologous transplantation (using my own blood stem cells) failed. But thanks to you, I could finally have a successful allogeneic stem cell transplantation using your blood stem cells, which was my last and only hope.

Now I am trying hard to live with a positive attitude. I know that I am still alive thanks to your stem cells as well as the support and prayers of many people. I promise that I will live my life to the full as a way to repay everyone.

Although I do not know your name, the job you do or anything else about you, please know that you are always on my mind and in my prayers. I cannot do anything for you directly, so I think the best way to return your favour is by helping those around me who are in need. And I will do my best to put others before myself.

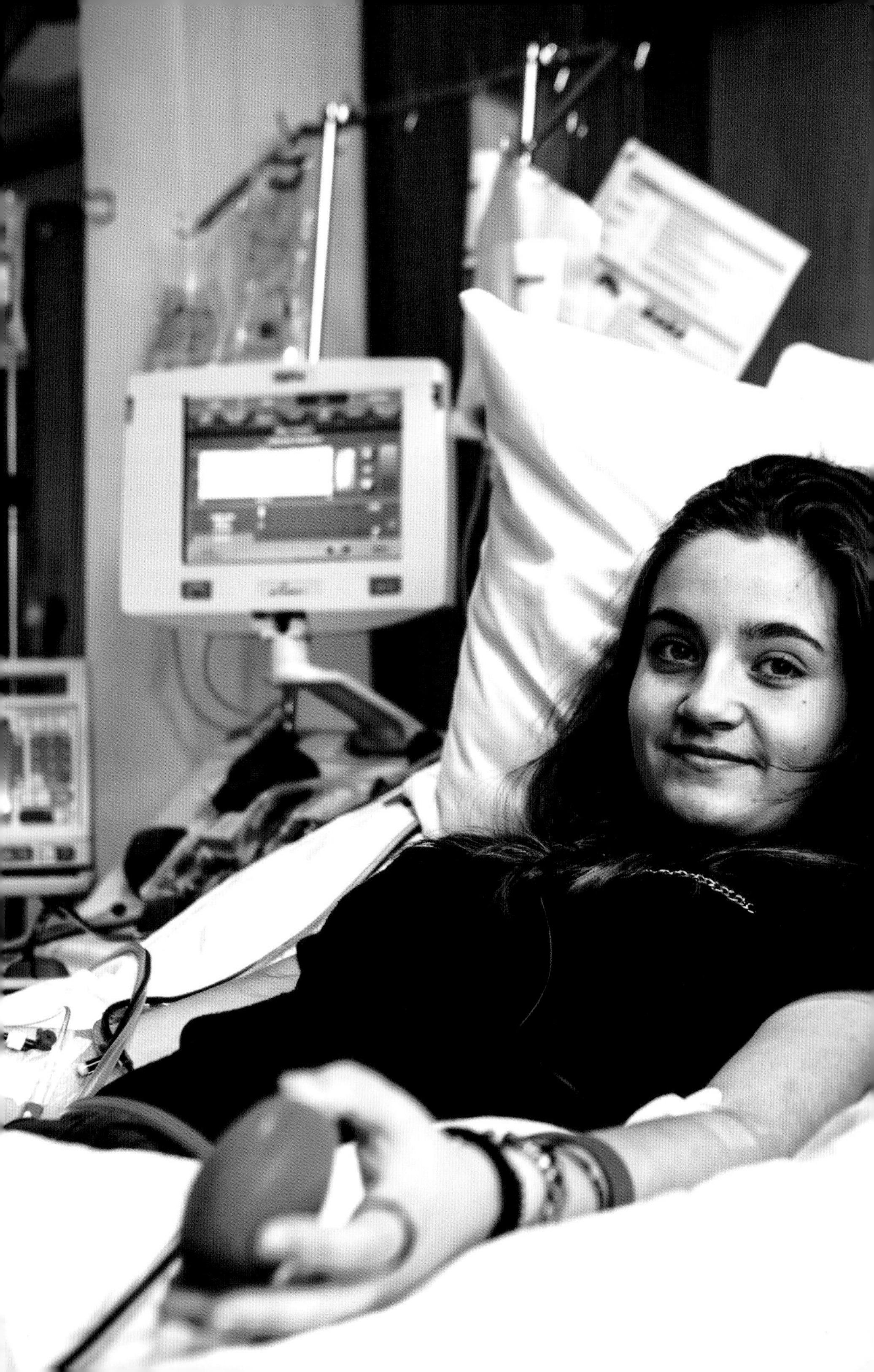

Section 3
The gift of giving

◀ The world's youngest stem cell donor at 17 (see page 133 "World's youngest donor")

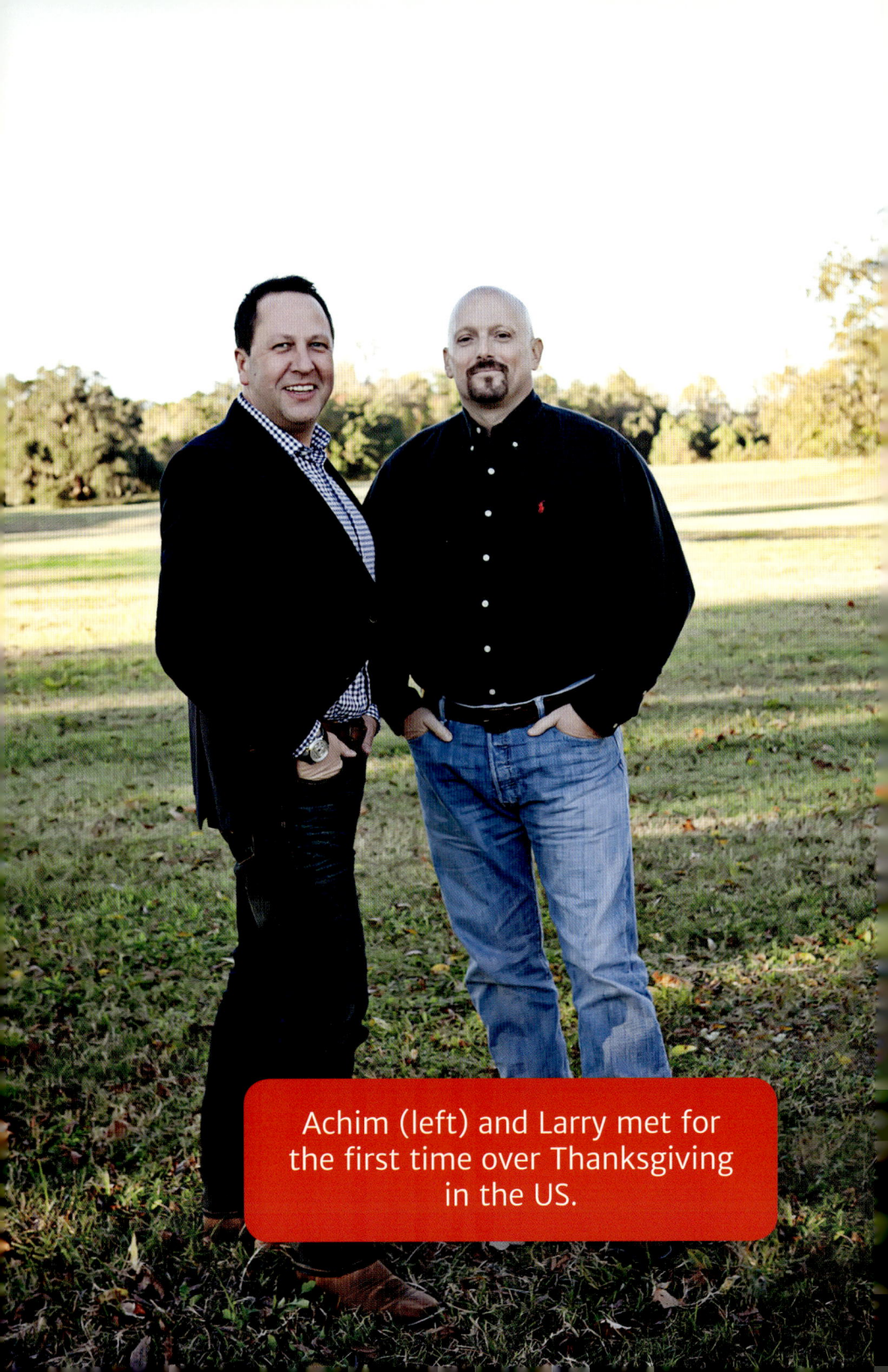

Achim (left) and Larry met for the first time over Thanksgiving in the US.

One match, two winners

Johann Achim Beissel, donated his bone marrow in 2011

It is strange that, although I have worked as a director at a large health insurance company for more than 20 years and have a pretty good idea of what blood cancer is, it was not until the spring of 2010 that I registered as a volunteer stem cell donor. A nurse at the University Hospital Muenster had been diagnosed with leukaemia and was looking for a match, so the hospital joined forces with the DKMS German Bone Marrow Donor Centre to organise a donor drive.

The registration process was extremely efficient. I just had to fill in a form and answer a few questions about my health. Then there was a small prick in my arm for the blood sample—something that is now done by simply taking a swab with a cotton bud. I helped myself to a quick coffee and sandwich at the free buffet, then headed home. With the exception of a letter confirming my registration, I did not hear anything else about it for almost a year. Then one day my mobile phone rang. When I picked up, a friendly voice from the DKMS told me that I was a potential match. My heart began to race. The DKMS asked if I would be prepared to donate. It was the easiest question I have ever had to answer—of course I was!

After some further testing to confirm that I was a suitable donor, I was told that I would have to donate via an operation. This would be a first for me. At the age of 48, I had been lucky enough to never fall really sick, and I had only been in hospital as a visitor.

The collection was initially scheduled for July 2011. But shortly before the big day, my contact at the DKMS told me the patient was not strong enough to go through with the transplant. The collection procedure was rescheduled for another date, which also had to be postponed. The DKMS asked if I was willing to wait. Of course I was. The patient's health was of utmost importance. I told them I was definitely still keen.

And then everything happened very quickly—so quickly that the hospital in Frankfurt where I had requested that the operation take place did not have a slot available, so I had to go to Dresden for the stem cells to be collected. The DKMS organised my flights and off I went.

I had been to Dresden many times on business, but this time it was as if I was looking at the city through a different lens. After taking a taxi to the hospital, I received a warm welcome and was shown to my room. Once I had settled in, I looked around the ward and realised how precious good health is. And how lucky I was to be in a position to help someone else become healthy again.

I slept well that night despite what lay ahead of me the next day and, before I knew it, I was lying on a trolley on my way to the operating room. I suddenly felt very anxious about the general anaesthetic. I saw the mask come down to my face, heard a little gas pass through the tube—and then I was out. It was like someone switched off the lights. There was no counting back from 10. I just fell asleep. After what seemed like five minutes, I woke up again. I had not felt a thing. The tube was out and the medical staff were smiling at me. That was it; I was a stem cell donor.

> Currently, around 80–90 per cent of Caucasian patients can find a matched donor for transplantation from unrelated donor registries worldwide. However, registries need to continually recruit new Caucasian donors to maximise the chances of patients finding the best match, and to replace their older donors with younger ones that may offer patients even better results with transplantation.

While I was coming around, someone asked if I knew who would be receiving my bone marrow. I was told that the patient was a 40-year-old American and that my bone marrow would be flying across the Atlantic. How great was that? Of course it did not really matter who would be receiving my cells—but it seemed such a coincidence given that I had flown to the US for a holiday just before my operation. And now, I had a permanent connection there.

Some time after that, towards the end of November, I sat down to write my first letter to the patient. I said that I hoped his transplant had gone well, and told him about my recent holiday to California. Christmas arrived and I thought about him a lot, wondering how he was doing. Then one day I came home to find a huge envelope from the DKMS in my letterbox. Hands shaking, I opened it and found my patient's response enclosed. But it was not just a letter from him—there were notes from his entire family. Even his dog said thank you with a paw print! I was very moved and suddenly felt an unbreakable bond with this family. This marked the beginning of two years of correspondence across the Atlantic.

> "But it was not just a letter from him—there were notes from his entire family."

As the end of the mandatory two years of anonymity drew nearer, it became clear that we wanted to visit each other as soon as possible. Because he was not yet allowed to take long flights, it was suggested that I make the first trip—I just was not sure where to. Two months before the end of the period of anonymity, I filled out a DKMS form with my details for the exchange. Then I received his information in my letterbox. His name was Lawrence 'Larry' Wilson Junior. A quick glance at his phone number told me that he lived in Texas.

I reached for the phone and dialled the number I had been given. After a few rings, someone picked up. I asked whether I was speaking to Larry Wilson Jr—I was. When I said that I was calling from Germany, the voice cried out, "Oh, you're my donor!" Because Larry had not yet received my details, I told him all about myself. We spoke on the phone for a good hour or so, then exchanged email addresses. The next morning, I woke up to find an email in my inbox from Larry's sister Fran. She wrote that the whole family had not stopped talking about me since I called the previous day. That she had cried with happiness and could not believe I was called Johann, because when they had found out that I was German, they had looked up common German names and decided to call me just that: Johann. Could that really have been a coincidence?

> "...they had looked up common German names and decided to call me just that: Johann."

After that we exchanged one email after another, and soon we had arranged my trip to Texas; it would be my first time in the US for Thanksgiving. In the meantime, DKMS had made contact with their American colleagues and asked if they could report on our meeting. Larry told me that local media were also interested in our story. A radio station, two newspapers and the biggest TV station in Texas wanted to interview us.

Although I had flown to the US many times before, this flight was special. As I waited to board the plane, I tried to imagine what it would be like when we met. What would I say? What would he say? I was so excited to get to Houston that it felt like we were flying more slowly than usual. Finally, after countless hours in the sky, the flight information showed me that we were close to our destination. After the airport formalities were completed and I collected my suitcase, I made my way towards the arrival exit. And then we saw each other.

Everything I had planned to say went out the window. It was just pure emotion—like we had known each other for years. Larry had already called me his brother in his letters, and I really felt like that at that moment. It was indescribable and I hardly noticed that TV crews were filming us. After a few quick interviews, it was time to head to Lake Jackson to meet 'mom and dad'. When we arrived, there was a large banner in front of the house that read, 'Welcome home, John'. And that was exactly how I felt; like I had come home. I had hardly climbed out of the car when Larry's mother, Christine, and father, Larry Senior, grabbed me in their arms. Fran was also there with her twin children Adam and Ashley. It was a wonderful moment.

After I had a quick shower, we sat down to eat. We talked a lot, cried many happy tears and shared plenty of laughs. I felt like part of the family. Larry was interested to know whether I had any allergies because there was a chance he could have the same ones now that he had my DNA. "Beer and steak," I joked in response. The look on his face told me that Larry and I had lots in common beyond my bone marrow!

> Haematopoietic stem cell transplantation involves transplanting the donor's blood and immune cells into the patient, which means the patient essentially acquires the blood-forming cells and immune system of the donor. Because of this, it has also been noted that patients will often acquire the allergies of their donors—including food allergies!

The next morning, I woke up to the smell of fresh coffee, bacon and scrambled eggs. We discussed our plans for the coming week over breakfast. Several appointments had been fixed: a radio interview, a newspaper interview, a football game on Sunday, horseback riding and, of course, Thanksgiving—complete with turkey and a TV interview. It was a packed schedule and our week together flew by.

By the time Thanksgiving arrived, Larry and I were well rehearsed at telling our story. All his friends and neighbours came over to meet me—his new 'brother'. Many of them could not believe that he would not have survived without my bone marrow.

While the turkey was roasting in the oven, a team from Houston's biggest TV station arrive with two cameras. Larry spoke about his illness and how happy he was that a donor had been found for him. And I spoke about how lucky I felt to have been able to help; how rare it is to get a chance to save another person's life. I also explained that donating bone marrow is a straightforward, painless process, even if an operation is needed. The key message we ended with was: go and get swabbed. It is so easy to help. And unlike organ donation, where there is usually one family left grieving, bone marrow donation is a win-win situation.

After mom Christine had made up a lunch box for the TV crew to see them off, we all sat down to enjoy our Thanksgiving meal.

Before I left to fly home to Germany, Larry and I agreed to visit one another as often as possible. I cannot wait to show my new brother and family my home country. And in the meantime, I have already booked my next visit to Texas: we will be celebrating my 51st birthday together on the Gulf Coast.

A unique gift

Craig Keller, Australia, donated his peripheral blood stem cells in August 2009

I registered with the Australian Bone Marrow Donor Registry as I felt it was something I could do to help others. Many of the people who donate stem cells do it for a family member who is in need of the product. I did not register for family reasons, but to hopefully be useful to someone else in the future. And sure enough, one day, I got a call saying I was a match.

I was definitely nervous about the extraction. But in the lead-up to it, I just kept thinking about the recipient and what he or she already had to go through while fighting cancer. At that time, the patient would be having treatment to kill their existing bone marrow, to get ready to receive my stem cells. So what I was going through was nothing in comparison.

In time I'll find out the status of the recipient and permit the release of my information so that we can be in contact. I'd encourage everyone to register as a donor. Who knows? One day you might even need the service yourself!

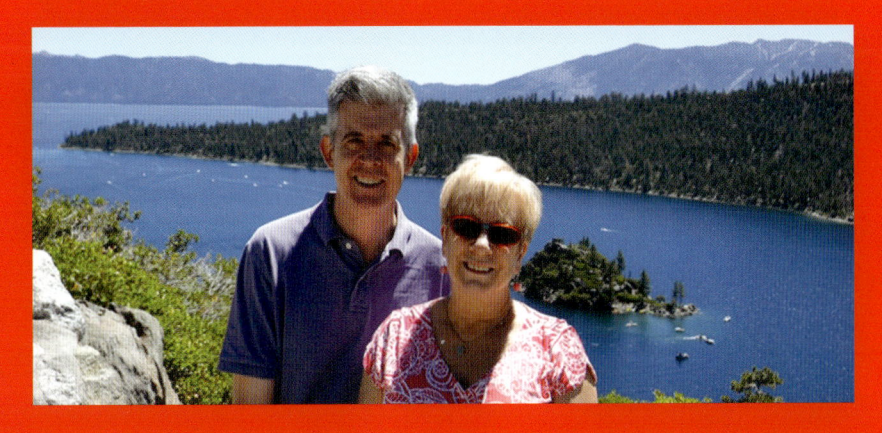

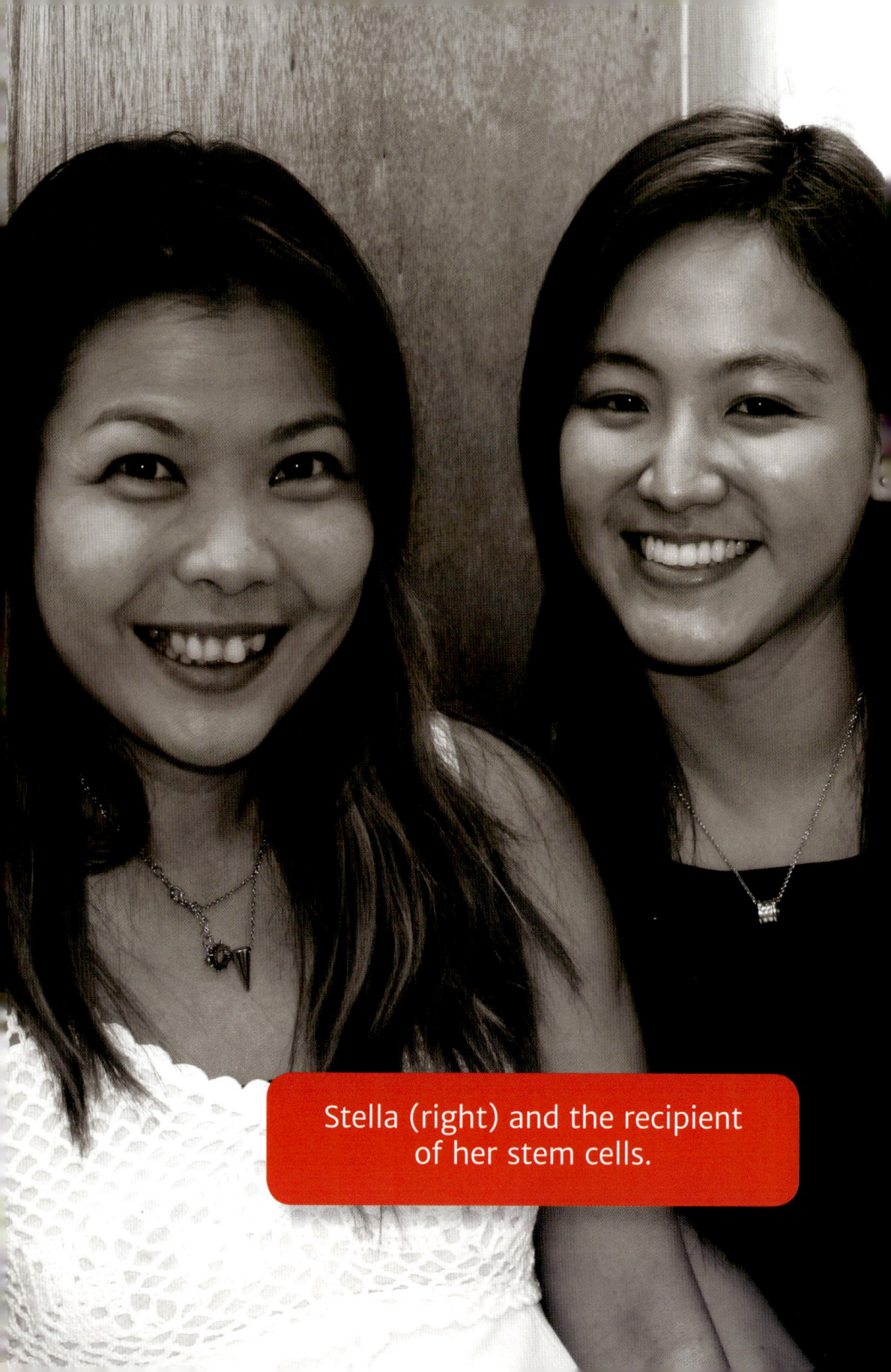

Stella (right) and the recipient of her stem cells.

A very special birthday gift

Stella Chua, Singapore, donated stem cells on her 21st birthday

A person's 21st birthday marks an important milestone in their life. It symbolises the transition to adulthood and maturity. It is also a day when that person hopes to receive gifts from their loved ones. However, I celebrated my 21st birthday by giving someone else a gift: a second chance at life.

Four years ago, when I was in my second year of studying nursing at the university, I donated blood at a local community centre. While I was there, some volunteers from the Singapore Bone Marrow Donor Programme approached me about registering as a stem cell donor. I agreed as I figured that the sooner I registered as a donor, the better the chance a patient might have to find his/her match.

I received a phone call six months later, telling me that I was a potential donor for a patient waiting for a stem cell transplant. I was incredibly surprised and felt honoured to have this opportunity to save another person's life. I remember exclaiming in joy to a friend who was with me at that time, "I am going to be a stem cell donor!"

Although I was not certain what the stem cell collection process was like, I was never afraid. However, when my family and friends heard that I was going to donate my stem cells to a complete stranger, they were in disbelief. Some even questioned my parents and discouraged them from allowing me to go through with such a 'dangerous' procedure.

Many people still have the misconception that stem cell donation is painful and life-threatening, which is not the reality today.

However, not even I—a student nurse—knew that stem cell donation could be done peripherally. When I met the doctor who was assigned to screen me and advise me on the process, I was expecting to have to donate through the traditional method of bone marrow extraction from my pelvic bone. And I was mentally prepared for it.

When I was told I could donate through the extraction of stem cells from my blood, I was very relieved. It also appeared to me to be a safer process with much less pain.

On my birthday, I underwent all the blood tests and investigations needed to make sure I was healthy enough to proceed. Thanks to the apheresis machine and excellent care from the nurses, everything went smoothly and my stem cells were successfully collected. The patient received them and, after initially battling a critical period of low blood counts, she recovered enough so that she could return home to her family. I did not know who she was, but I continued to pray for her good health.

> A traditional bone marrow transplant is performed under general anaesthetic, with the bone marrow extracted from the donor's pelvic bones. This marrow contains blood-forming cells—otherwise known as haematopoietic stem cells (HSCs)—which produce white blood cells that fight infection, red blood cells that carry oxygen and platelets that help to stop bleeding. These blood-forming cells may also be able to help fight some cancers.
>
> In the 1980s, researchers found that these HSCs could also be extracted from the blood flowing in peripheral blood vessels. These peripheral blood stem cells (PBSCs) are coaxed out of the bone marrow when the donor is given a drug called G-CSF. The PBSCs can then be extracted through apheresis—a procedure where the patient's blood is extracted by a machine that separates the different blood fractions by centrifugation, retaining the white blood cells that are rich in stem cells, and returning the rest of the blood to the donor. Donors can undergo this procedure as an outpatient.

By complete chance, I got to meet the recipient several years later at the annual Survivors' Reunion Party at the hospital where I was working. When the transplant coordinator told me the recipient wished to meet me, I was overcome with excitement. I could feel my heart pounding. Then, the moment we were introduced, my tears began to flow. I wept as I held her hands and looked at the healthy woman before me. Her hair was long, her body strong, her skin radiant and her smile wide. No one would ever have been able to tell, just by looking at her, that she was a leukaemia survivor.

> "When I was told I could donate through the extraction of stem cells from my blood, I was very relieved. It also appeared to me to be a safer process with much less pain."

I have since gone on to become a fully-fledged nurse trained in oncology and haematology. Being a bone marrow donor has helped to shape me into who I am today. The gift I gave on my 21st birthday was not only for the recipient—it was also a gift for me: a memory that I will treasure forever.

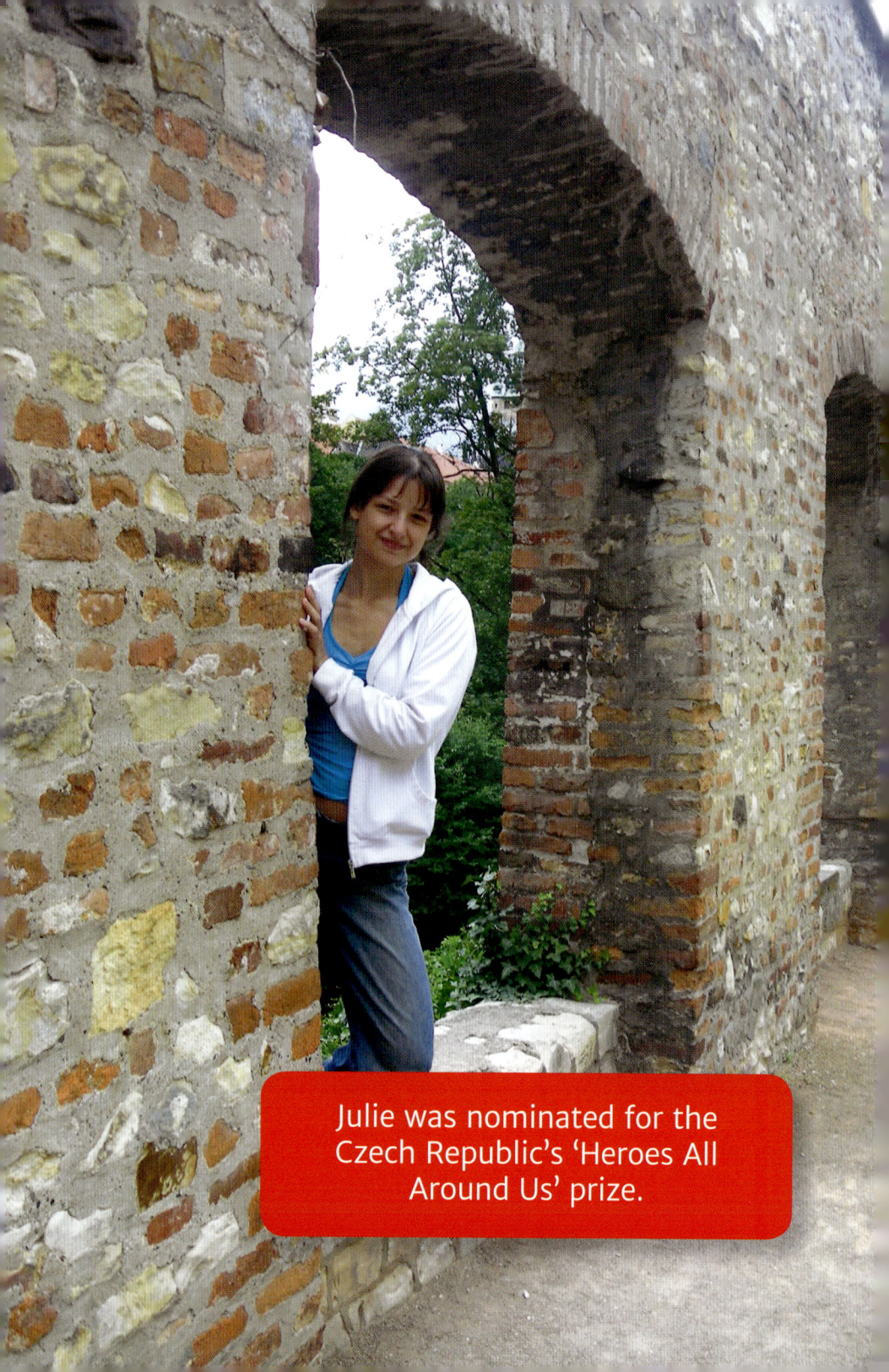

Julie was nominated for the Czech Republic's 'Heroes All Around Us' prize.

Finding Julie

Lucie Marckardt, Coordinator at the Czech National Marrow Donors Registry

Tracing a donor for verification typing is something we deal with many times a day. But there was one search that turned out to be very different from any other.

It sometimes happens that registered donors do not pick up our phone calls or reply to our letters. Sometimes their email addresses do not work, or we do not have their email address on file. But on this occasion, the donor—a young woman called Julie—was answering her phone but not saying anything. So we called again. And again. Still nothing but silence. We were puzzled.

> "Finally, you have sent me a message! I am hard of hearing and cannot communicate by phone. Please email me."

We decided to try one last thing before closing the search and informing the patient that the donor was not available; we sent Julie a text message on her mobile number. To our surprise, she replied almost immediately: "Finally, you have sent me a message! I am hard of hearing and cannot communicate by phone. Please email me."

The mystery was solved. We had no records of Julie's hearing problems as they had developed over time. But she did not hesitate in agreeing to proceed with verification typing. Julie ended up donating her stem cells and saving our patient's life.

Since that successful transplant, Julie has gone on to be nominated for the national 'Heroes All Around Us' prize, which honours people who have demonstrated outstanding bravery. In addition, she was featured on the cover of the magazine that we distribute twice a year to all our registered donors. However, Julie still does not see that what she has done is a big deal—that, in spite of her disability, she went out of her way to save the life of someone she had never even met.

Finding Julie reminded us all that there is a very thin line between success and failure, and between life and death. Sometimes it pays to be persistent.

When a person registers as a volunteer donor with a bone marrow registry, a blood or tissue sample is taken to determine their tissue type using a process called human leukocyte antigen (HLA) typing. A person's HLA helps their immune system determine whether a cell in their own body belongs to them or someone else.

In bone marrow transplantation, HLA typing is important in establishing the precise tissue type and identifying the best matched unrelated donor—ensuring that the immune systems of both the patient and donor are as compatible as possible. When a patient needs bone marrow, a donor search is performed among registries around the world for a donor that matches the patient's HLA type. If a potential donor is found, the donor's HLA is tested again (verification typing) to make sure that they really are a match.

Virtue, not duty

Dr Mihran Nazaretyan, Medical Director, Armenian Bone Marrow Donor Registry

When you hear the word 'donate', what do you think of? Most picture money, food or perhaps even blood. But did you know that a bone marrow donor can give blood stem cells that can permanently cure patients with fatal blood diseases?

I was moved by what one of our stem cell donors said one day. Frederic, a stem cell donor from Tehran, Iran, who gave his blood stem cells through the Armenian Registry to save a Belgian woman, told us, "Many people I have seen since my stem cell donation have said how brave I have been. A few others have said how careless I have been... But I don't think either bravery or madness comes into it. Even if the discomfort were considerably more than I underwent to donate, I would do it again..."

What Frederic said reminded me of Immanuel Kant's classic ethical work on the *Foundations for the Metaphysics of Morals* (1785). His

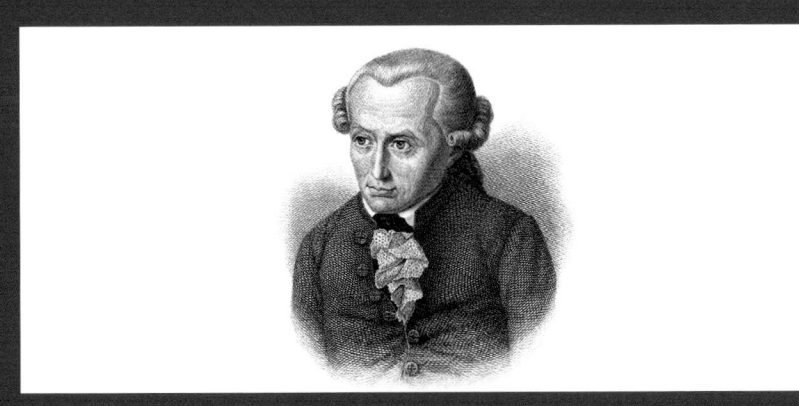

Immanuel Kant

moral formulae were derived from a duty towards humanity and pure reason. He believed that only actions performed for the sake of duty have any moral worth, and that the more we desire not to do something that we perhaps have a duty to do, the higher the moral worth becomes. Conversely, if we perform an action just because we are inclined to do so, it holds little moral worth. This theory would suggest that the moral rightness or wrongness of donating stem cells or bone marrow goes beyond 'sake of duty' and therefore holds up a higher moral standard.

But Frederic's story of altruism is not the only one. There are many others, such as that of Vahe, a young man from Yerevan, Armenia, whose blood stem cells were found to match a young Italian girl with a form of blood cancer. Through Vahe's gift of blood stem cells, the girl is now in remission. These two have become firmly connected with one another, even though they never met each other in person or made any form of direct contact. Today, they continue exchanging cards with blessings for each other, and share their life events and successes.

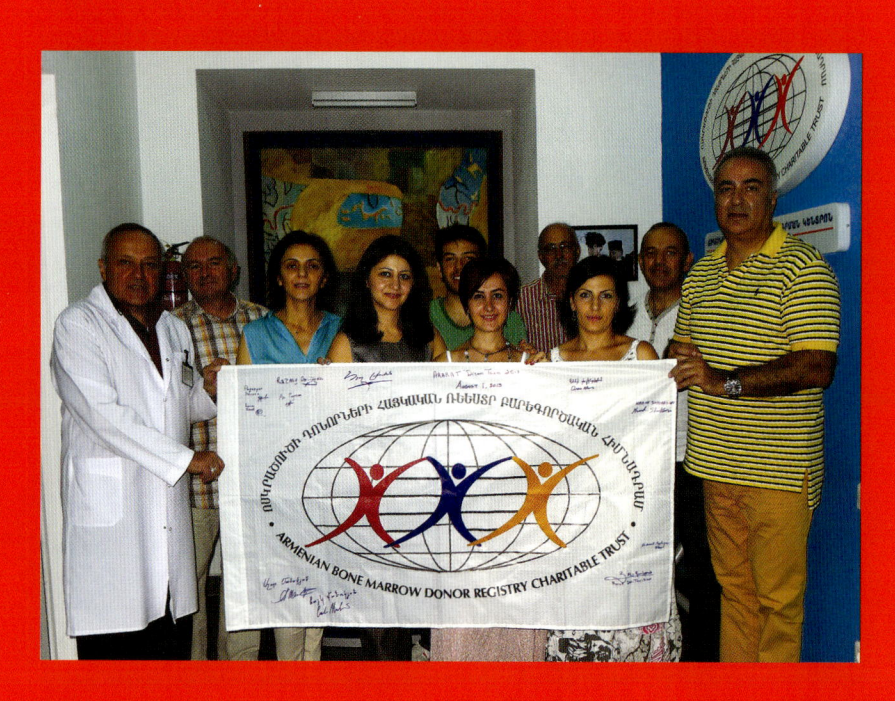

Frederic and Vahe—two men of virtue who helped others to overcome their fatal diseases—represent the best qualities and 'giving' philosophy of any human being. I believe that a life lived through receiving is fortunate, but a life lived through giving is a blessing.

> "Virtue never stays lonely. It is bound to have neighbours."
> Confucius, 551–479 BC

做对的起自己
良心的事

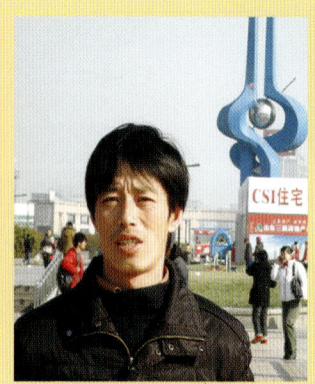

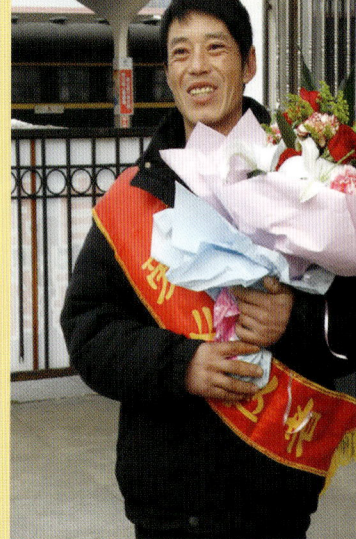

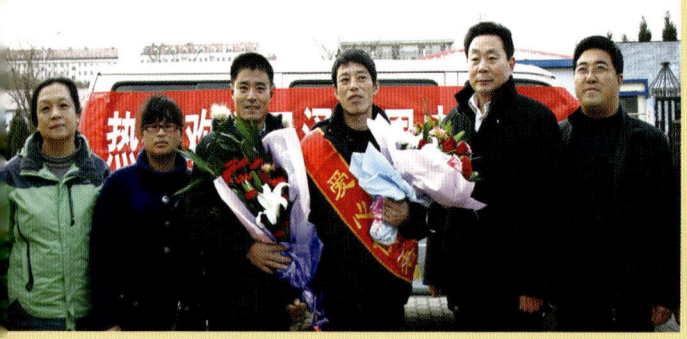

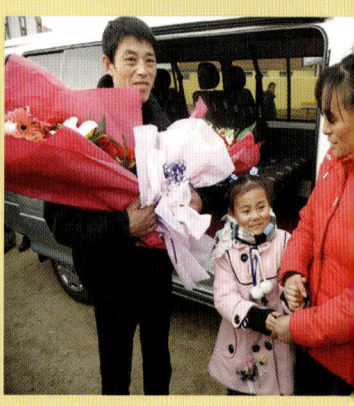

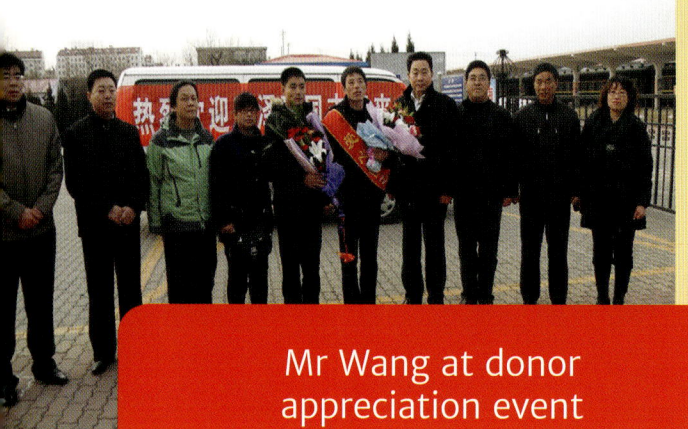

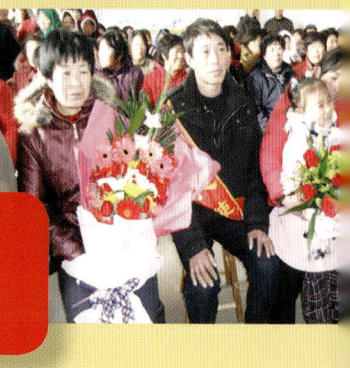

Mr Wang at donor appreciation event

A family affair

Contributed by Lu Zhaoxia and Sun Yijing, China Marrow Donor Program

When the Red Cross launched a haematopoietic stem cell donation drive in 2007, a man named Wang Zejian voluntarily registered and donated a blood sample. In May 2010, the Red Cross notified me that Wang Zejian was a preliminary match for a patient. He did not hesitate in agreeing to donate upon receiving the call.

Once we got news that the subsequent high-resolution typing had also been successful, Wang decided that it was time to inform his family. He thought that they would be supportive, as they usually were of his decisions. However, unexpectedly, both his wife and mother objected to his donation, and his wife even threatened to divorce him! Wang was faced with a dilemma. On the one hand, there was a patient out there waiting desperately for a transplant. On the other hand, Wang now faced strong opposition from those closest to him.

The main concern for Wang and his family was the donation's potential adverse side effects. So I decided to continue engaging them and handed Wang the phone numbers of former donors, hoping that he would be able to gain more insight from them. My manager and I also decided to visit Wang and his family in person. When we arrived at their village in Rongcheng, we met Wang's mother. She appeared to be a down-to-earth old lady whose only concern was her son's health. Although we provided a detailed description of the procedure to try to dispel her fears, she left the room muttering her disapproval. The situation had reached a stalemate.

Some weeks later, when we had nearly given up hope, I received a call from Wang. He sounded very stressed. Although he had not yet managed to persuade his mother and wife, he was aware that the patient's condition did not allow for any further delays. So he had decided to donate his stem cells at the hospital in Jinan without telling his family. I was sorry that he did not have the support of his family, but was relieved that he wanted to proceed.

> "To make matters worse, his younger brother and sister-in-law were on their way to Jinan to look for him. But Wang's conviction was never shaken; he knew that he was doing a good deed in saving a life, and that he had to proceed."

On the day of the procedure, Wang acted like his usual self to avoid arousing any suspicions. Once he had arrived safely in Jinan, he received a call from his family. Wang thought that, as he was already preparing for the donation, his family members would not argue with him—so he told them the truth about where he was.

Upon hearing the news, his wife immediately raised her objections. Facing opposition from his wife and his mother, and receiving persistent phone calls from the rest of his family as they tried to dissuade him, Wang wept. It seemed like no one could understand his conflicting feelings. To make matters worse, his younger brother and sister-in-law were on their way to Jinan to look for him. But Wang's conviction was never shaken; he knew that he was doing a good deed in saving a life, and that he had to proceed.

Once they arrived at the hospital, Wang's younger brother and sister-in-law had a long discussion with the doctors in charge of the transplant. They came to understand that the stem cell donation was safe for Wang and essential in order to save the patient's life. Wang was moved to tears when his younger brother finally gave him his blessing.

After the donation was complete, Wang called home to let them know that he was well. His wife and mother cried with joy when they heard his familiar voice. His unwavering spirit moved them deeply. In fact they were so moved that they were inspired to follow in his footsteps; one year later, his wife, brother, sister-in-law and 10 other villagers donated blood with the Red Cross.

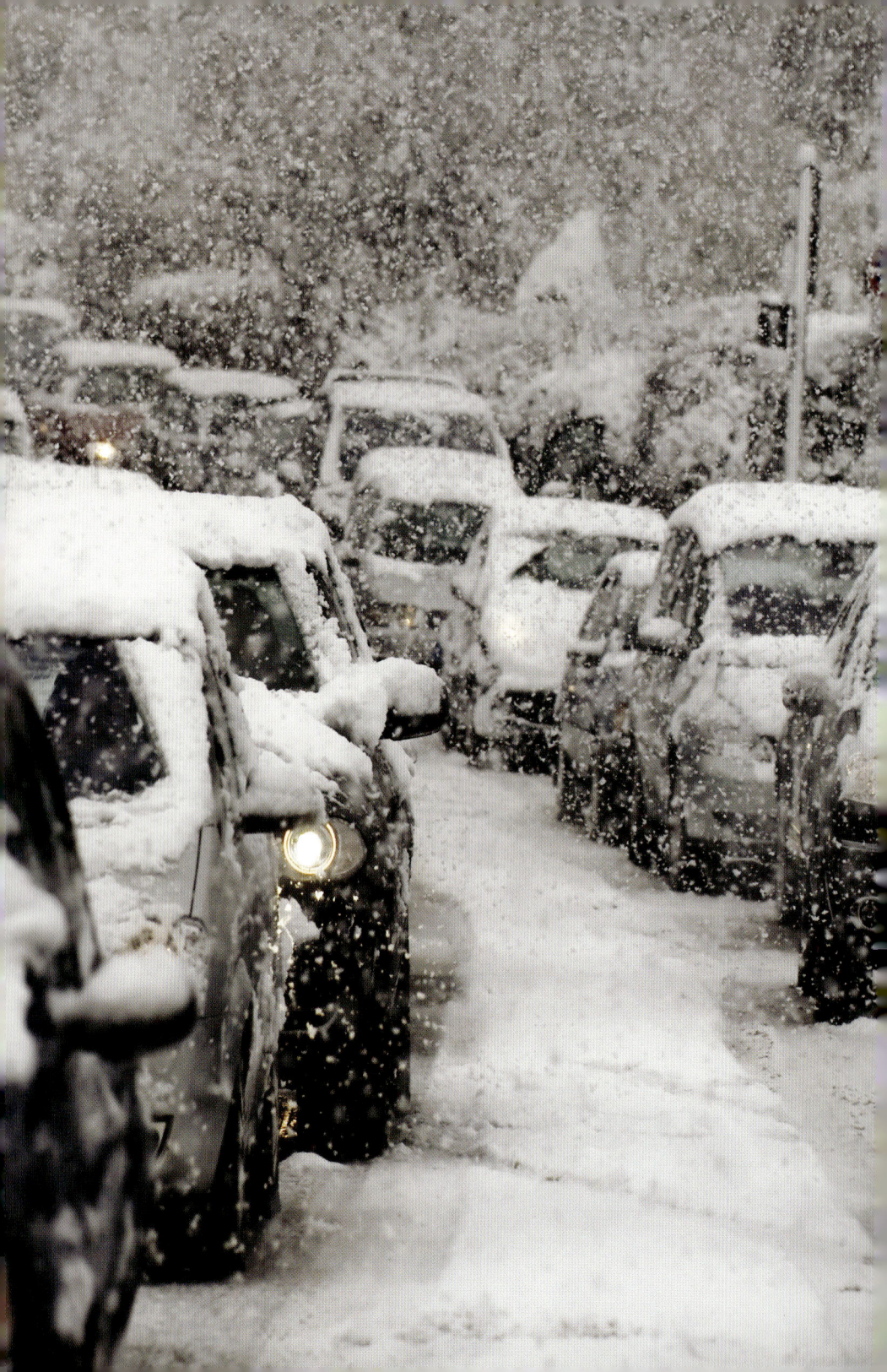

The journey

Markus Ranker, donated his stem cells in 2009

Written with the support of Sabine Hildebrand, Head of Global Donor Recruitment, DKMS

Just one month after registering as a volunteer donor with DKMS, I heard that my tissue characteristics had been matched with those of a patient. After I had undergone further medical examination, an appointment was made for me to donate my stem cells on 21 December 2009 at the University Hospital of Dresden.

DKMS organised the entire trip to Dresden for my girlfriend and myself, making sure it would be as convenient and comfortable as possible. Our flight from Cologne was booked for the day before the procedure so I could arrive in good time before my appointment and get settled in. However, Mother Nature had different ideas. On the day of our flight there was heavy snowfall, and by 11 am, air traffic had come to a halt at many airports in the region.

Despite reassurances from airline staff that our flight would take off as scheduled, none of the planes arriving at Cologne were ours. The clock continued ticking into the night, and at 9 pm we finally received the news we had been dreading—our flight had been cancelled. I was still determined to donate. After all, someone's life depended on me. But it was impossible to reschedule my appointment at such short notice, as the transplant procedure had already started for the patient!

We looked into taking the train, but many train connections had also been cancelled due to the bad weather. At that point, we were informed by the DKMS team that another donor was in exactly the same situation as I was. After a few phone calls, we met up with

Christoph, the donor, and his wife. We discussed our options—how about renting a car? Unfortunately, we were not the only ones with this idea; there were plenty of others already waiting in line for a rental car. A sense of desperation began to take over. Then Christoph suddenly remembered that a friend of his brother owned an SUV. That friend was quick to respond and did not hesitate to agree to lend it to us.

It was not long before Christoph's brother pulled up at the airport, bearing hot tea and some thick blankets. Finally, at midnight, we began our 500 km drive through the night from Cologne to Dresden. The journey was long and we were all exhausted, but no one slept. We were all anxious about whether we would make it in time.

After a long drive and with over half the distance covered, we were just starting to believe we might make it when the traffic ground to a halt. There was an accident on the road ahead of us. After everything we had been through, I could not believe our bad luck! We still had 170 km left to cover and only three hours to do it.

> "...we were just starting to believe we might make it when the traffic ground to a halt."

We decided to tell the police on site about the importance of our trip. The police officer in charge did not hesitate to guide us up the emergency lane. After clearing the accident, we were able to continue on with our journey.

When we finally arrived at the collection centre in Dresden, just after 8 am, I felt as if a huge weight had been lifted. What a relief! A quick snack and a warm drink later, Christoph and I were hooked up to the machines that collected our stem cells. After all the trouble we had gone through to get to the clinic, I was pleasantly surprised to discover that the donation process was pain-free. Just two hours later, my stem cells were ready to go on their own trip—hopefully one without any snow delays!

The journey to Dresden taught me that, while the road to achieving your goals may not always be smooth, the obstacles encountered can make success taste so much sweeter. I have never regretted going the extra mile for the person who has received my stem cells, whoever he or she might be. I would not hesitate to do it all over again.

> When a patient needs a bone marrow donor, transplant centres will not only search the local bone marrow registry, but bone marrow registries around the world. When a donor is found, the collection of the stem cells usually takes place at special centres with staff trained in performing collections from healthy volunteer donors. These generous and selfless donors may be from any part of the world, and will sometimes go to extraordinary lengths to make sure they can donate in a timely manner to save a life.

Saranya, after she had donated her stem cells

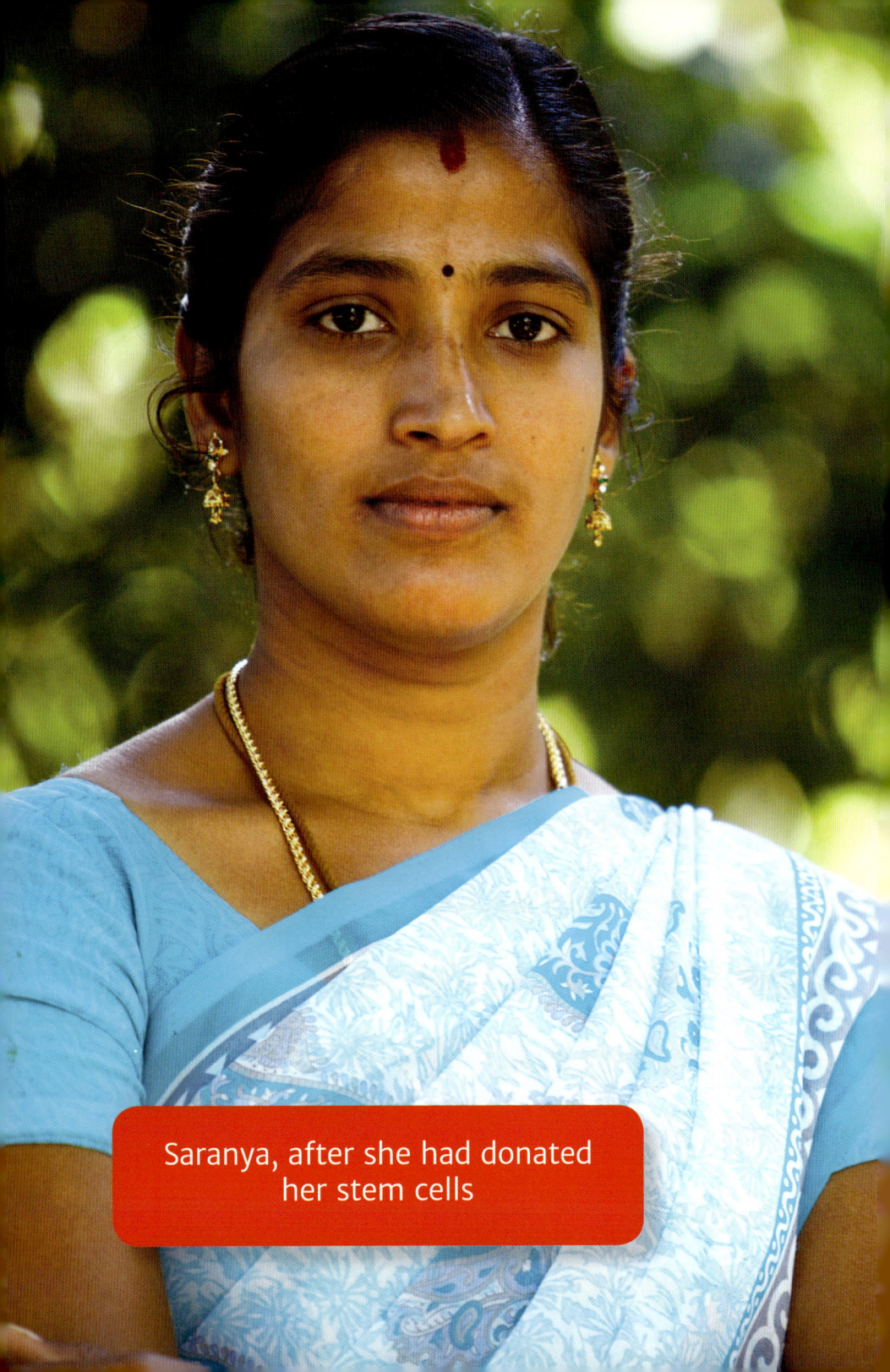

Passion and perseverance

Contributed by Raghu Rajagopal, Co-founder and CEO, Datri Blood Stem Cell Donors Registry, India

Bodinayakanur is a small town in the state of Tamil Nadu in India, with a large community of people descending from this town living in Florida in the US. One member of this US-based community, a 26-year-old woman, was suffering from a form of blood cancer. A local college in Bodinayakanur was chosen as the location for her donor drive. I was at the drive in March 2010 and we recruited around 200 donors, all young men and women who were students at the college.

Sadly, no match could be found for this patient from Florida, and she passed away without a transplant. But in July 2013, we found a match for a 10-year-old boy who was suffering from a fatal blood disorder—a 24-year-old woman who had signed up at our original drive in 2010.

We tried contacting the potential donor using the details that had been given on the application form, but we were unsuccessful. Through a series of phone calls, I managed to get hold of the college's board member who had initially approved the drive. When I spoke to him, he said he was happy to help us locate the donor.

I selected two people to go to the town and assist with the search: Sudhir, a Datri employee, and Ravi, who runs a travels company and is also a Datri volunteer. It took them around nine hours to reach the town from Chennai, which is where we are based.

When they arrived at the college, Sudhir and Ravi looked through the old records to see if they could find the donor based on her graduation year. It was then they discovered that the donor's brother, who had also studied at that college, had recently died. They found the donor's address and decided it was best to visit her in person.

When they knocked at the door of that address, a lady opened it. She was the donor's mother. She had tears in her eyes—not only had she recently lost her young son, but her daughter (our donor) had eloped with a boy from a different community against her parents' wishes. They had no idea where she was. Sudhir and Ravi sympathised with them and began making enquiries with neighbours, but they could not get any information as to where the donor was living with her new husband.

During his conversation with the potential donor's parents, Sudhir deduced that the donor's husband either drove a small truck or an auto rickshaw. So they set out to talk to drivers around town, asking after the donor's husband. Sadly, that search did not yield any results.

Sudhir and Ravi began to lose hope and wanted to return to Chennai. I spoke with them over the phone and explained that I still had hope. I was certain that if we could locate the donor, she would donate, as her actions had already proven that she was ready to make important life decisions—like getting married to someone from a different community, against her parents' wishes. I asked them to stay in town a while longer and check into a local motel, then wait to see if they heard any more news.

The next day, they went to a local lawyer referred to them by the college. The lawyer suggested they walk the streets and knock on people's doors to get more information. You only hear about these door-to-door visits happening at Halloween in the US!

Although it was unusual, the idea paid off. By chance, they knocked on the door of a lady who turned out to be the grandmother of the donor's husband. She told them that he now worked on a farm and lived in a hilly region nearby, but she did not know his address. Sudhir and Ravi set off in search of them. After a few more enquiries—there were several farms on the hills surrounding the donor's home—they finally found the donor! Sudhir and Ravi were overcome with joy.

The donor's name was Saranya, and her husband was called Thangam. After Sudhir explained how Saranya had the opportunity to save the life of a 10-year-old boy, the couple were convinced that she needed to donate her stem cells.

However, Thangam's parents were also very conservative and were against the idea of letting their daughter-in-law travel to Chennai and undergo the procedure. Thangam advised them to get the opinion of a local doctor. Fortunately, the doctor they met with had practised in developed countries, and so was familiar with the process and managed to change their minds.

> "If you are passionate and continue to persevere, you can save lives!"

The donation could finally go ahead. Without wasting any more time, Sudhir and Ravi accompanied Saranya and Thangam, as well as Thangam's brother and sister-in-law, to Chennai. (The couple did not want to go to the big city without at least two family members.) Once they arrived in Chennai, all the necessary testing and preparation processes—from verification typing to collection of the blood stem cells—were completed in a record two weeks. Now, more than a year after the transplant took place, the young recipient is doing well and is already back in school.

The moral of this story? If you are passionate and continue to persevere, you can save lives!

Leticia and her father

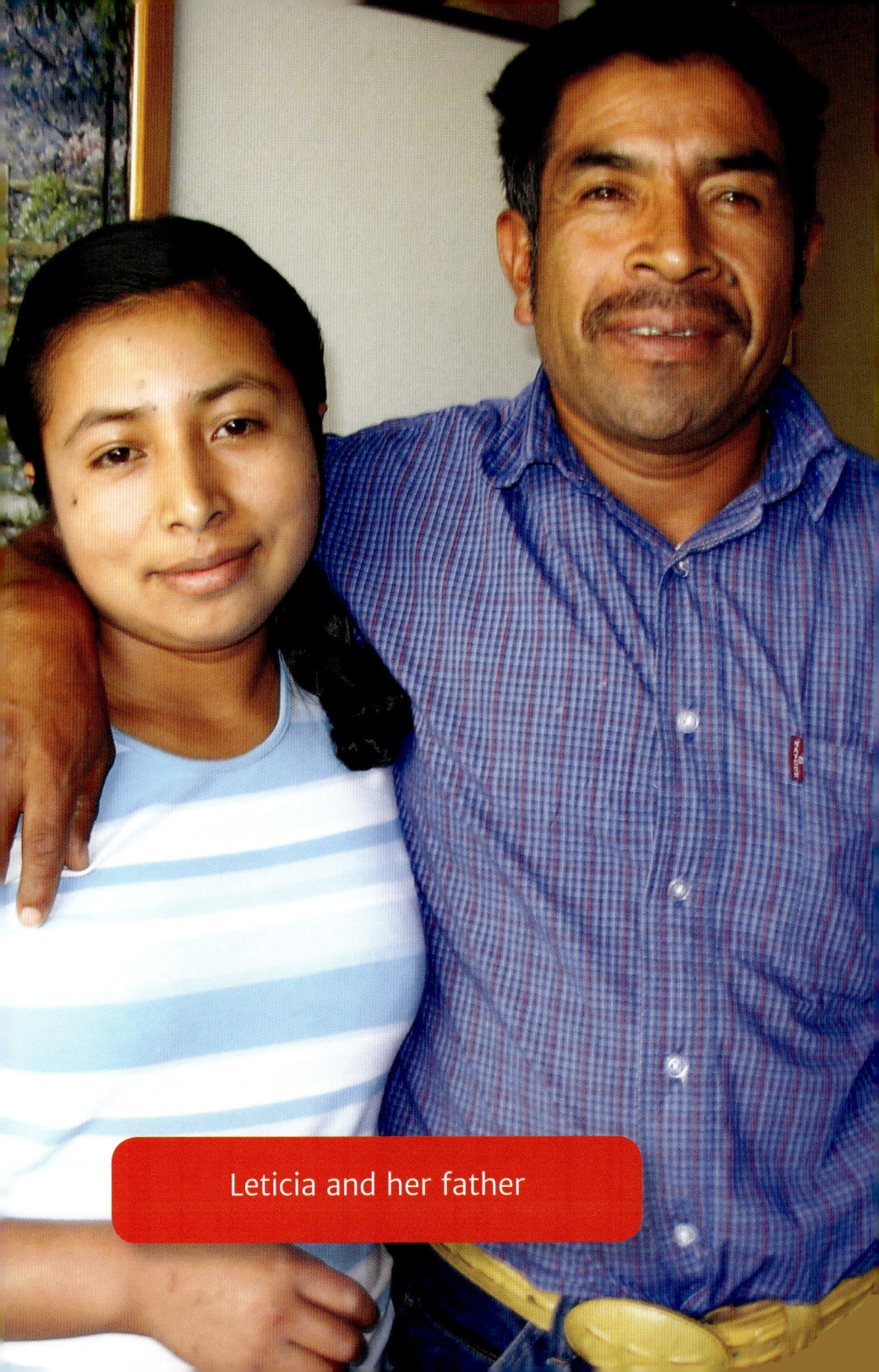

The kindness of strangers

Prof Dr Clara Gorodezky,
Director of the Mexican Bone Marrow Donors Registry (DONORMO)

One August, we received an email from a minister at a church in Fontana, California. He told us the story of a father and daughter who needed help getting from Chiapas state to Mexico City because the daughter was potentially a match for a member of his church requiring a bone marrow transplant. These two people were Don Ignacio and his daughter, Leticia López.

Around a year before, the patient in question had left the town of Margaritas in Chiapas to pursue the American dream. He wanted to join one of his brothers and work in Fontana so that he, too, could support his family back home. However, just 12 months later, the new immigrant began to feel sick and weak. Soon afterwards, he was diagnosed with acute myeloblastic leukaemia.

Members of the patient's church in Fontana realised that his situation was very uncertain. They cared for him while a haematologist at one of California's best cancer hospitals offered to begin the patient's chemotherapy treatment at no cost.

The doctor and the church leaders contacted our team at DONORMO and provided us with all the information we needed to be able to start a donor search in Mexico. We coordinated with the lab in Chiapas to arrange for blood samples to be sent to us here in Mexico City. After we had confirmed that 18-year-old Leticia was a compatible donor, she and her father travelled to the US Embassy in Yucatán to file for a humanitarian visa. Sadly, their request was denied.

By that time, the church in California had also contacted the authorities for help, pleading with the Mexican consulates in both Washington DC and in San Bernardino. However, they were also unsuccessful.

Fortunately, a few weeks later, the physician treating the patient in California received compassionate aid from the US government and was informed that the patient would be covered by state medical insurance. We were immediately asked to perform the necessary HLA typing, and begin the workup and arrangements for the product to be transported. The Mexican government, via the Secretary of Integral Development of the state of Chiapas, funded the plane tickets for Leticia and her father to travel to Mexico City.

When they arrived, Leticia was undernourished, had anaemia and was generally in poor health. We had to bring her back to full health before we could proceed with any possibility of a donation. Speaking in her native Tzotzil language, Leticia insisted that she would not leave Mexico City without fulfilling her mission of giving life to another human being.

It took more than one month to treat Leticia until she was well enough to go ahead with the donation. During this time, all of us at DONORMO, the church in Fontana and the medical team at the patient's hospital worked together closely to make sure that everything went to plan, and that Leticia and her father received the best possible care.

> "The donation was a success … Leticia and her father will never forget this once-in-a-lifetime experience."

The donation was a success and, afterwards, the product was accompanied by a courier to the US. Meanwhile, Leticia and her father returned home to the Tzotzil people in the Sierra of Chiapas—but I am sure they will never forget this once-in-a-lifetime experience.

Sascha (left) with Raphi before his donation.

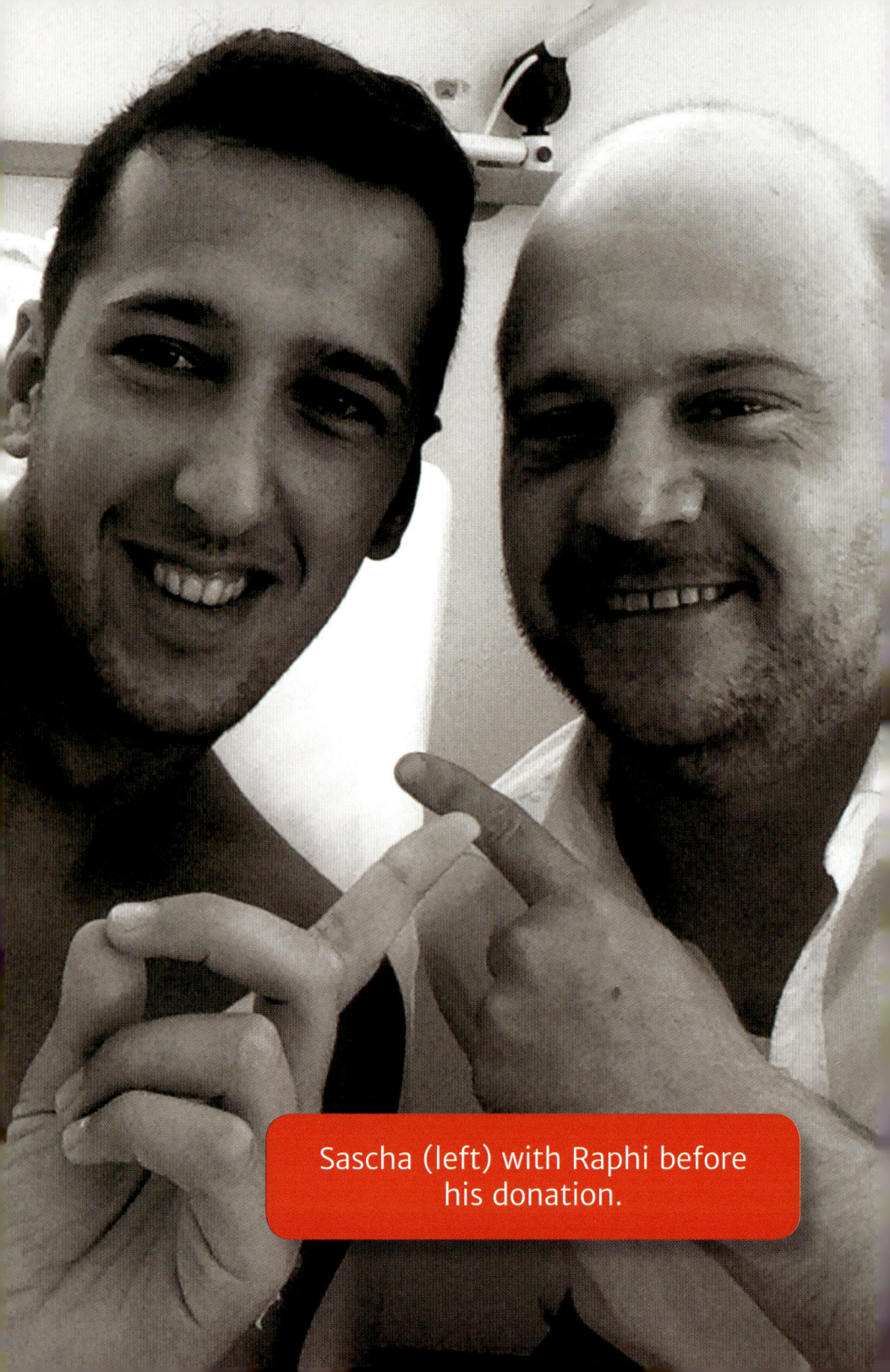

A chance meeting

Sascha Fischer, Switzerland, donated his stem cells in 2013

I first heard of hyperleukocytosis several years ago when I learned that my good friend Raphi was suffering from the disease. Although I was familiar with the term leukaemia, I did not understand at the time what it would mean for my friend, or for his family or future.

While the search for an unrelated compatible donor for Raphi was ongoing, a group of his closest friends organised a public call for blood and blood stem cell donations. I got involved in that, along with a dozen other people, and registered as a blood stem cell donor myself. Unfortunately, no donor could be found for Raphi at first.

The feeling of being unable to help him haunted me so much that I decided to donate blood regularly and, in that way, give back at least a small portion of the good fortune that being healthy entails.

> Hyperleukocytosis is a condition where there are too many circulating white blood cells. These excess cells can cause problems in the blood circulation and, when the condition is severe, it can be life-threatening. Leukaemia is one of the main causes of hyperleukocytosis and, if the leukaemia is found to be a high-risk type, a bone marrow transplant could be the only cure.

Then one day, five years after I had registered as a blood stem cell donor, I received a call from the transfusion centre in Basel. I was told that I was a potential match and was asked if I would still be willing to donate. After being properly briefed and some careful consideration, I decided to proceed. I would donate my blood stem cells through an operation on my pelvic bone.

Two weeks later, it was time for my operation. Just as I was checking into the university hospital in Basel, something incredible happened. I ran into my old friend Raphi—the very person who had inspired me to register as a donor five years before. That coincidence dispelled any remaining fears I had. I was suddenly 100 per cent certain that I was doing the right thing.

The donation went so well that I was able to return home just two days later, and go back to work shortly after that. It is a great feeling to know that someone has been given a chance at a better life, maybe even a healthy life, because of what I did.

From China with love

Zhang Jiansheng
Zhang Jiansheng, physician at Laiwu Hospital of Traditional Chinese Medicine and a stem cell donor

Submitted by Lu Zhaoxia, China Marrow Donor Program

I felt it was a great honour to become the first unrelated donor in Laiwu to successfully donate haematopoietic stem cells. What impressed me most was the concern shown by the staff at the Red Cross Society of China, the Bureau of Health and the hospital before and after my donation, as well as the concern of my colleagues. This made all my efforts worthwhile.

Nian Yixin
Nian Yixin, Shandong province, China, donated his stem cells in 2014

Submitted by Lu Zhaoxia, China Marrow Donor Program

I am someone who lacks confidence. I often feel that I am not a very capable person. But having successfully saved another life with my own blood, I now feel that I am at least of some use.

Generous donor
Mr Chen Chuanyong, China, registered as a donor with the China Marrow Donor Program in September 2008

Submitted by Yang Wanli and Jiang Yaping, China Marrow Donor Program

I still cannot believe that my HLA has been matched with three different patients on three separate occasions. The first time was in

2009. I felt it was my destiny to donate and looked forward to doing it as soon as possible so that the patient could recover from his terrible disease. But I then received news that the patient could not go ahead with the transplant. I was a little disappointed, and very worried for the patient. I felt uneasy and concerned for a long time afterwards.

On hearing that my HLA had been matched a second time, I was very happy—but worried that it would fall through, just like it had during the first occasion. To stop myself from becoming too emotionally involved, I did not ask any questions about the recipient. All I knew was that they lived in Hangzhou in eastern China. Following the advice of the Red Cross, I focused my attention on staying in good health. I felt that my life no longer belonged to me alone; another person depended on it too. I waited anxiously but, regrettably, this transplant was also called off.

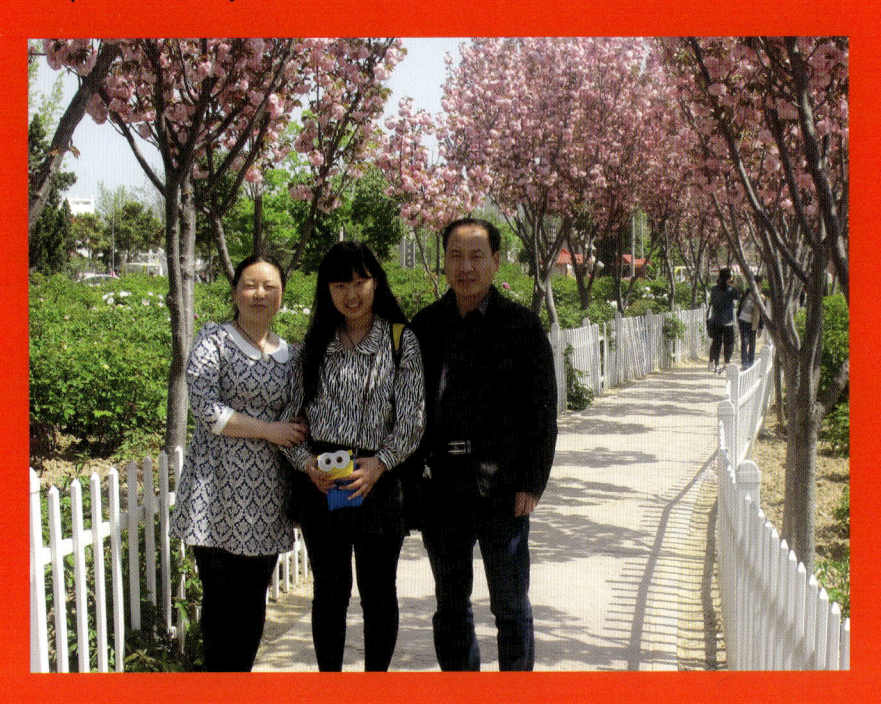

On the third occasion, I was finally admitted to the provincial hospital for an injection of G-CSF after several months of preparation. The stem cell mobilisation procedure was tough. I couldn't sleep and experienced back pain. But the thought that I could save someone's life helped to relieve my discomfort. The following day, as the collection was underway, I was given the sad news that the recipient had already passed away. I had almost grasped his hands and saved his life. But all I could do now was shed tears for this stranger whom fate had brought so close to me.

After the procedure was over, I donated the compensation that donors usually receive for absence from work to the patient's family. That poor family was tortured by the loss of their loved one, and in my mind it was the only way I could express my condolences. My thoughts are still with them today.

Jeff and Kim

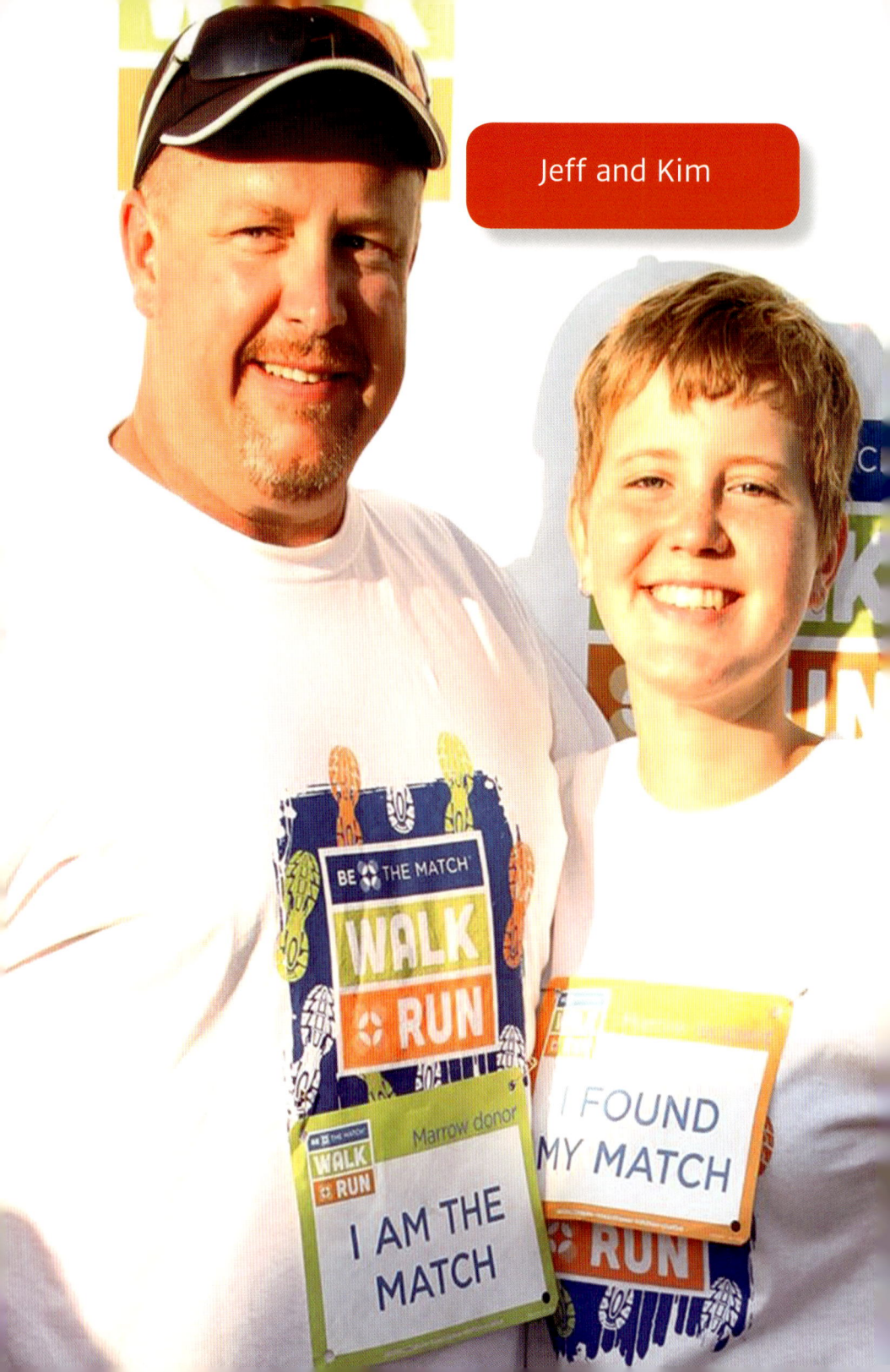

A birthday surprise

*Jeff Haertling, National Marrow Donor Program/
Be The Match volunteer and donor*

Like many people, I signed up as a stem cell donor because I had a friend in need. It was 2007 when a colleague asked me to sign up in an attempt to save her daughter's life. With a simple cotton swab on the inside of my cheek, my DNA was collected and then stuffed into an envelope along with some personal medical history and my contact information.

My DNA was then decoded and recorded in a laboratory somewhere, but unfortunately it was not matched to my friend's daughter. Sadly, no matched donor could be found for her in the global database of blood stem cell donors. She lost her battle to leukaemia six months later.

After that, I all but forgot about the registry until my phone rang a few years later. A nurse from the National Marrow Donor Program/ Be The Match was calling to tell me that I was a perfect match for a 16-year-old girl who was fighting blood cancer. I had kids of my own, and I knew what the child's parents must have been going through. As such, my decision to go ahead with the donation was easy. During the course of the year, as I had a surgical procedure to extract my healthy stem cells and transplant them into this teenager, something else magical happened. Although I had been asked to help save her life, the experience also changed mine.

One of the conditions of the transplant process is a one-year period of anonymity. This is to protect both the donor and recipient should the worst outcome occur. So my recipient and I called each other 'Marrow Mates' and wrote cards to one another through the registry, under these names. I would try to lift her spirits when she needed it, while she helped me see the world through a fresh pair of eyes.

At her very young age, my 'Marrow Mate' had already faced the gravity of a terminal illness. Having lived most of my life without such a heavy burden, her words and experiences gave me a new perspective.

During those 12 months, we exchanged 27 anonymous letters. After the one-year mark had passed, my phone rang again. This time, it was the recipient's parents, who were calling on behalf of their daughter. We laughed, then cried, and laughed some more, before coming up with a plan to surprise my 'Marrow Mate' the following weekend. Not only would Kim be celebrating her first 're-birthday' post-transplant, but it was also a special one—her 18th.

> "Through the perfect fusion of science, fate, good fortune and miracle, my marrow donation gave Kim a second chance at life—and changed my life forever."

A few days later my wife and I flew to Kim's hometown, rented a car and drove straight to a restaurant for dinner. Once arrived, we were seated at a specially designated table. As we ordered our drinks, a family was seated opposite us. Sitting a mere four feet away from me was a now cancer-free young lady, who had just been handed a birthday card from her parents that contained the name of her donor. "He lives in St Louis and is waiting for your call," it read. As she dialled my number and placed her cell phone on speaker, both her phone and another nearby rang in unison. She looked around, puzzled. After the second ring, I answered—and my salutation of 'Hello' echoed throughout the dining room. Kim turned around, then screamed with excitement as I approached her with my arms outstretched. It was a hug that I'll never forget.

Through the perfect fusion of science, fate, good fortune and miracle, my marrow donation gave Kim a second chance at life—and changed my life forever.

Our families now visit each other as often possible. Be The Match holds an annual 5K walk/run event to promote donor awareness, and I have travelled to Portland twice to take part in the event with Kim. Flying 2,000 miles to be able to walk three miles with my 'Marrow Mate' is incredibly rewarding.

Today, Kim is a sophomore in college and living every day to the full. While she is still catching up on the couple of years that leukaemia stole from her, she has also chosen to give back by volunteering at the hospital where she was treated, and by promoting the National Marrow Donor Program/Be The Match whenever possible.

I have chosen to do the same—by volunteering at local donor drives, speaking at colleges and church groups about joining the registry, and trying to dispel the myths associated with the donation process. Next to my family, supporting Be The Match and its network of international registries will be the focal point for the second half of my life.

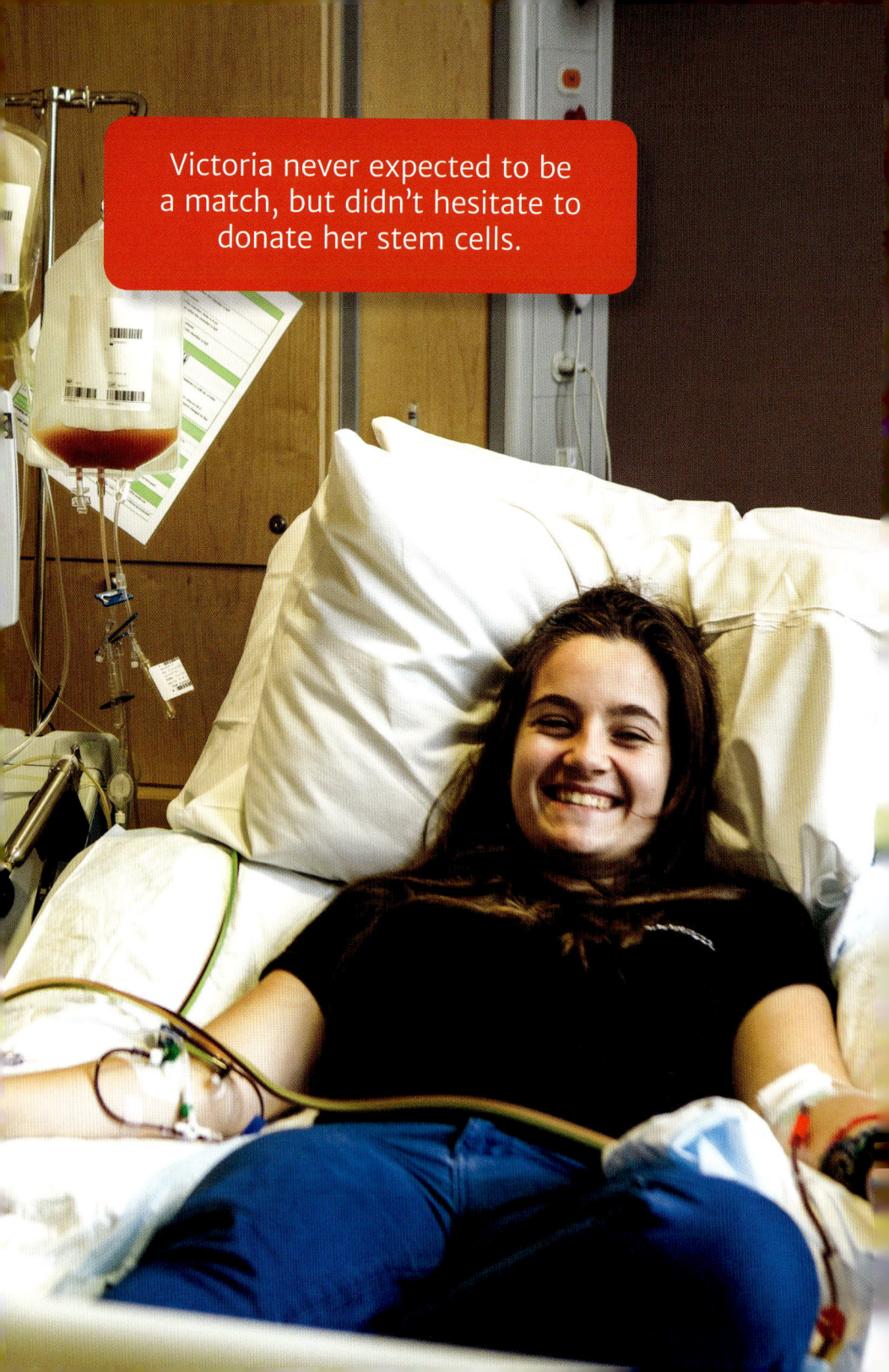

Victoria never expected to be a match, but didn't hesitate to donate her stem cells.

World's youngest donor

*Victoria Rathmill, from Macclesfield, UK, became the world's youngest stem cell donor at the age of 17.
She signed up at 16, and donated in November 2013.*

*Written with the support of Jo Badger and Emma Radway
–Bright at Anthony Nolan.*

Some people from Anthony Nolan came into school in October 2012 and gave a presentation about how some people who are very ill need stem cell treatments. I thought, "I'll sign up as a donor when I'm 18; I'm probably not going to make a difference anyway." But then a family friend developed leukaemia and it hit home how serious diseases like these were.

I signed up as a donor a few weeks later. I sent off a saliva sample but, for some reason, my sample did not want to cooperate, so I had to send a blood sample as well. It was March or April by the time I could be placed on the register. After that I just did not think about it. I did not expect to get a phone call within six months of signing up. The whole incident was just relegated to the back of my mind. At the beginning of October 2013, I received a text asking me to ring Anthony Nolan. I was in a history class, so for the rest of the class I was panicking because I more or less knew what it was about.

> While most countries require a donor to be at least 18 or 21 years of age, some do allow younger donors to donate, depending on the country's minimum age for a person to give legal informed consent.

The first person I called was my mum. Then I phoned Anthony Nolan. The woman I spoke to said I might be a possible match, and asked whether I would be willing to send a blood sample. I just said, "Yep, that's fine."

I did not have to think very hard about it. I had the chance to save someone's life. I was not expecting to have this opportunity, and I was a little scared, but I was excited for what it meant.

First I had to go down to London for a medical exam to make sure I was fit and healthy. I went on my own, which was my first time in London without other people accompanying me. My dad, Tony, got the London Underground map out and worked out exactly where I needed to go. I was happy to go on my own—it gave me a little peace and quiet for the day. And I even managed to fit some shopping in!

> "Donating is not as difficult as you expect it to be and not as bad as some people make out. So as long as you do not have a phobia of needles, you will be fine."

All I would say to other people is that you should definitely sign up as a donor. Even if you get the call, you can always back out, but donating is not as difficult as you expect it to be and not as bad as some people make out. So as long as you do not have a phobia of needles, you will be fine.

I would like to meet the recipient of my stem cells one day. If they write me a letter I would be happy to write one back, but if they do not, that is okay too. I just hope they are getting better and that I have helped—that is the most important thing.

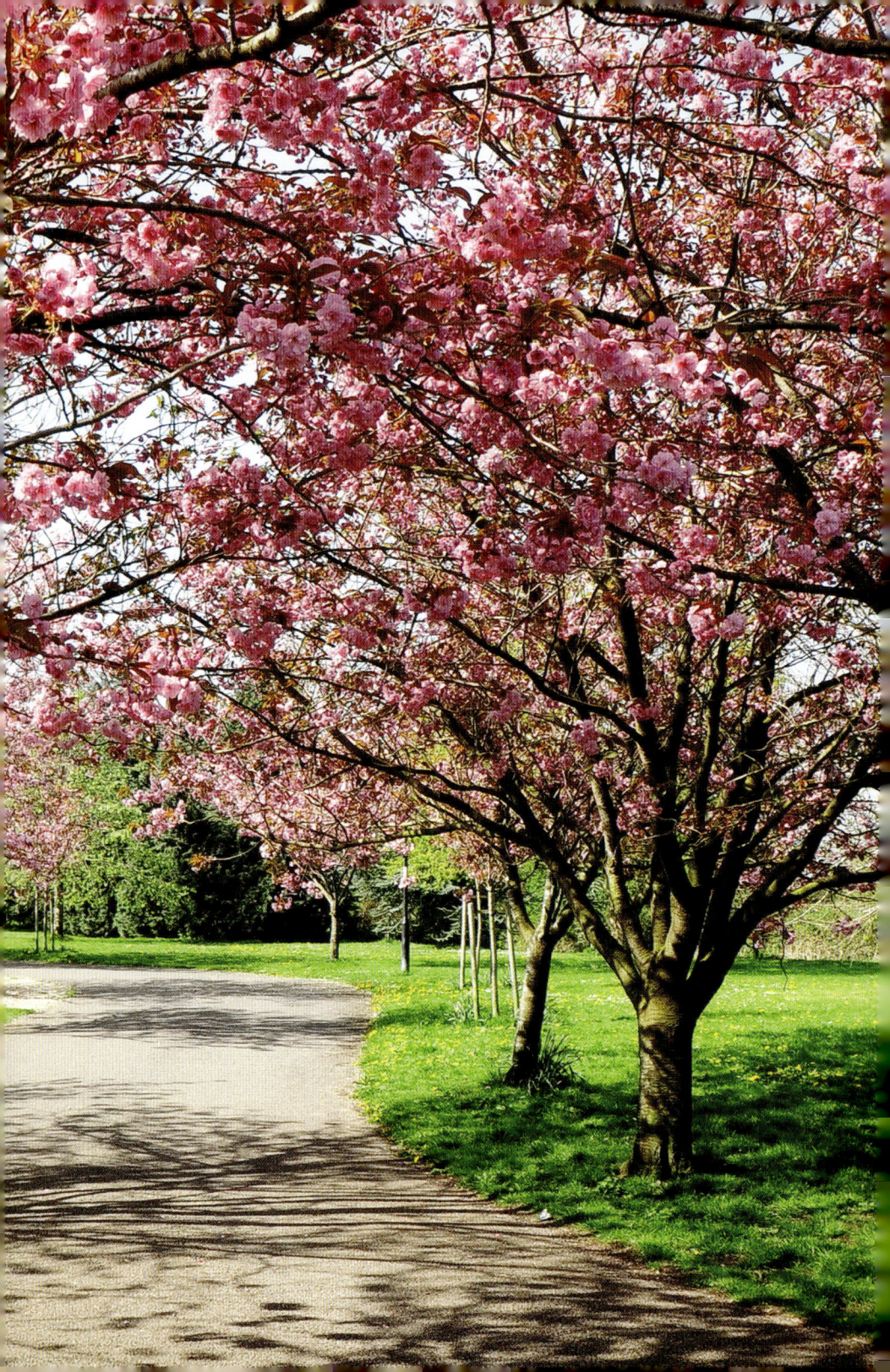

Happiness and gratitude

Kim Dong Wook, South Korea, donated his bone marrow in 2009

It seemed as though I had suddenly fallen asleep. When I awoke, a coordinator from the Korea Marrow Donor Program was by my side, watching over me with a soft smile. "It won't be long until the blood extraction is finished," she said. During the procedure, I could not move my arm properly, so I was feeling a bit stiff. But when I thought back over what had happened over the past three months, my discomfort seemed like no big deal.

Three months ago, I was busy with my work in the office when I received a call from an unknown number. "This is the Korea Marrow Donor Program. A few years ago you registered as a stem cell donor, is that right? I'm calling because we have a patient whose genotype matches yours. Are you still willing to donate?"

I called my wife and told her about the situation. And just as I had predicted, my wife did not have any objections to me going ahead with the donation. Of course, she was a bit worried, but more than that, she was concerned that something might happen to the patient in the three months leading up to my donation date. "Shouldn't it happen sooner?" she asked.

The results of my final genetic test and health tests were good. As the donation drew closer, I began to feel an enormous sense of duty. The coordinator told me about my responsibility as a donor not to change my mind or get sick, because from now on the patient would be preparing for the stem cell transplantation.

> "Seeing the eyes of my youngest daughter fill with tears as she waved at me from the window of the taxi, I suddenly felt a big lump in my throat. But then I thought, "If I am feeling like this, how must the patient's family be feeling?""

Finally the day arrived. Late one Sunday afternoon, I was admitted to hospital for three days for my blood to be extracted. My wife and children accompanied me to support me. My children, who saw their father wearing a hospital gown for the first time in their lives, were extremely anxious. I told them, "Don't you worry. Daddy is not sick, but there is a boy who is very sick and daddy is going to give a bit of himself to help him. Daddy will be coming home soon."

Seeing the eyes of my youngest daughter fill with tears as she waved at me from the window of the taxi, I suddenly felt a big lump in my throat. But then I thought, "If I am feeling like this, how must the patient's family be feeling?"

The extraction started the next morning. I had the luxury of a single room to myself, so I could spend my three days at the hospital in a relaxed manner, watching TV and reading books.

Seeing the bright red pack of blood once the extraction was finished, I was overcome with emotion. I wondered how eagerly the patient's family must have been waiting for it. And I prayed that my stem cells would be of great help to them.

A little later on, I decided to give the patient, whom I knew was a teenager, a gift: a basketball. I jotted a few lines on a card telling him to see the ball as a sign of hope and that he should recover quickly so he could play a game of basketball with me one day. And after some time, I received a reply from the patient's mother through the coordinator.

Her letter read: "Ten years ago, I lost my eldest son to a brain tumour. And then my youngest son was diagnosed with leukaemia. But fortunately, our prayers were answered, and a few months ago we received the wonderful news that a donor was found whose genes matched our son's. That was a day of both happiness and gratitude."

While reading this letter together with my wife, we shed many tears. My wife told me: "Darling, you have done a really good thing. If you did not do it, you would have regretted it for the rest of your life." Nowadays I always keep this letter in my bag—and whenever I am going through a tough time, I take it out and remind myself how fortunate I am.

When I tell people that I donated my stem cells, most pat me on the back and ask if it was a painful experience. I think that more positive publicity is needed to inform people that being a donor is not at all dangerous and donating is rarely very painful. My stem cells provided a lifeline for a patient. But I also feel that I have learned many things that I could not have learned anywhere else. I have grown as a person.

Every day, I pray for the full recovery of this child, who is, even now, fighting his disease.

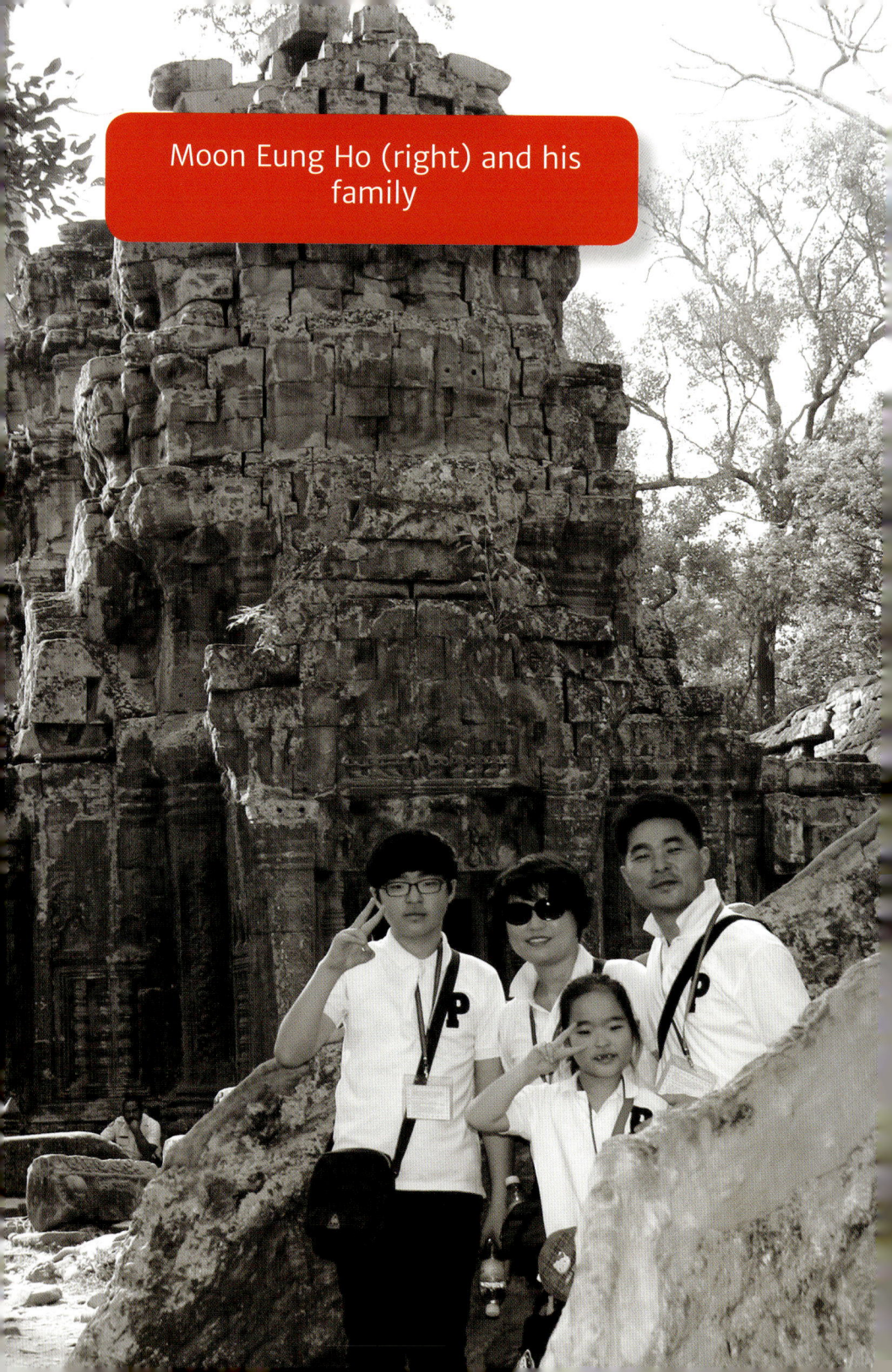

Moon Eung Ho (right) and his family

Third time lucky

Moon Eung Ho, South Korea, donated his bone marrow in 2008

I work as a teacher at Osan High School in Gyeonggi Province, South Korea. Every time I am assigned a new class, I remind my students that: "Love is shown in your deeds, not in your words." In 2008, I was given the ultimate opportunity to practise what I had preached.

That summer, I received a phone call from the Korea Marrow Donor Program informing me that my genotype had been matched with that of a leukaemia patient—a young girl who was only 10 years old. I had previously been contacted by the program on two other occasions in 2004 and 2006. Then I had also chosen to donate, but unfortunately could not because of the poor health of one patient and because my genotype was not a 100 per cent match with the other. Because of these experiences, I promised myself that I would definitely agree to donate if I had the chance again.

> "Love is shown in your deeds, not in your words."

But that was easier said than done! Although I wanted to donate immediately, this poor child developed some inflammation in her mouth, so the donation process had to be postponed. As a father and teacher, I was very worried about her and felt great sympathy for her parents. Because her immune system was weak, it took their daughter a long time to recover from an inflammation that any healthy person would have recovered from in a week.

Finally, after many twists and turns, I went into hospital in the winter of 2008 to donate my stem cells through peripheral blood transfusion. The day that my blood stem cells were extracted also happened to be my birthday—and it's a birthday that I will always remember.

I stayed in hospital for four days. As I walked home after being discharged, I felt so excited. This was the most meaningful thing I had ever done in my life. When I arrived home, my wife, our young son and our daughter gave me a warm welcome. My son told me that I was the best and gave me a thumbs-up. Even now, he is proud of the fact that daddy saved somebody's life by donating his bone marrow.

I hope that, by setting this example for my children and my students at school, I will encourage them to be more considerate when they grow older. I want to teach them that, above all, we should cherish, love and care for others.

No longer strangers

Mr Liu Wentao, Shandong province, China, donated his blood stem cells in 2013

Submitted by Lu Zhaoxia, China Marrow Donor Program

One year has passed and I wonder how the patient who received my haematopoietic stem cells is doing. Is she well enough to go out? I don't even know her name. I only know that she is one year older than I am and has a seven-year-old son. If it were not for the stem cells that connect us, we would never have known each other existed. Now, my blood runs through her veins and we are no longer strangers.

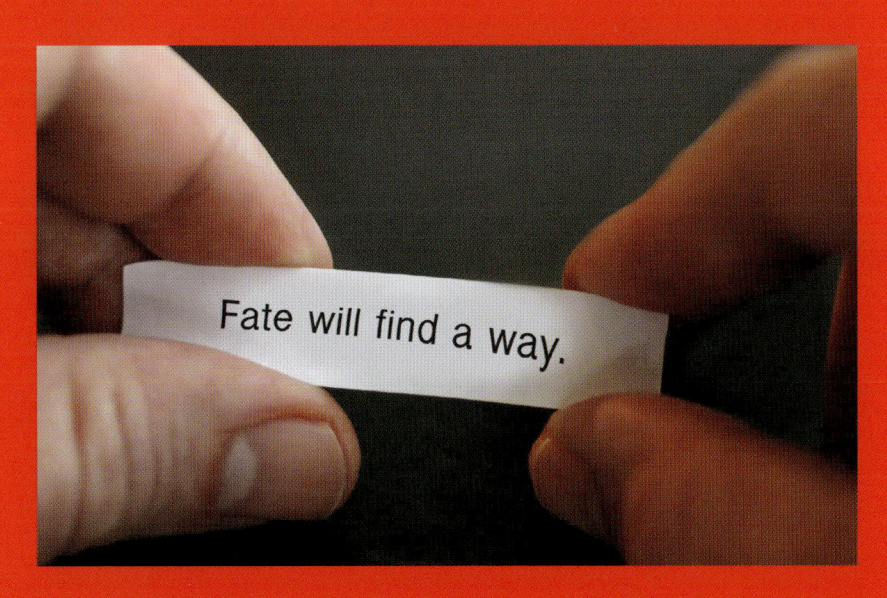

In China, we believe in fate. I was the only one among millions of volunteers whose stem cells were a match for hers—isn't that destiny?

> "In China, we believe in fate. I was the only one among millions of volunteers whose stem cells were a match for hers—isn't that destiny?"

It was back in my university days when I felt the urge to become a donor. One day I was watching a television programme that showed a young leukaemia patient reading a book. The narrator said the child would die soon if a stem cell donor could not be found for her transplant. Staring at the screen, I suddenly felt that the white sheets and white walls of the hospital were horrifying; not a place where this lovely child should die. The programme moved me deeply. In the following months, those images appeared repeatedly in my mind and eventually spurred me to sign up as a donor.

Around a year later, my phone rang and I was told that my HLA type was a preliminary match with a leukaemia patient's. I was very keen to donate my stem cells to save a life, but I had to persuade my family members to agree with me. After all, I was no longer a carefree bachelor, but a husband and father. Although haematopoietic stem cells are harvested from peripheral blood and the whole procedure is quite safe, my mother strongly objected. She has many traditional beliefs that are difficult to reason with.

As the collection day drew nearer, my mother still would not agree with my decision to donate. I decided to call my brother and ask him to distract our mother by inviting her to visit his new home in southern China. That way, she would not be around when I went for my procedure.

Later on I discovered that she was well aware of my ploy, but chose not to reveal that she knew of it as she realised she could not stop me from going ahead with the donation. My mother may be a stubborn woman, but she has a very kind heart.

My stem cells were successfully collected under the excellent care of the staff at the hospital and the Red Cross Society of China. My wife accompanied me and stayed with me throughout the collection. Seeing me lying on the hospital bed, she turned away to dry her eyes. I could see love and affection shining through her tears, and I knew then how proud she was of me.

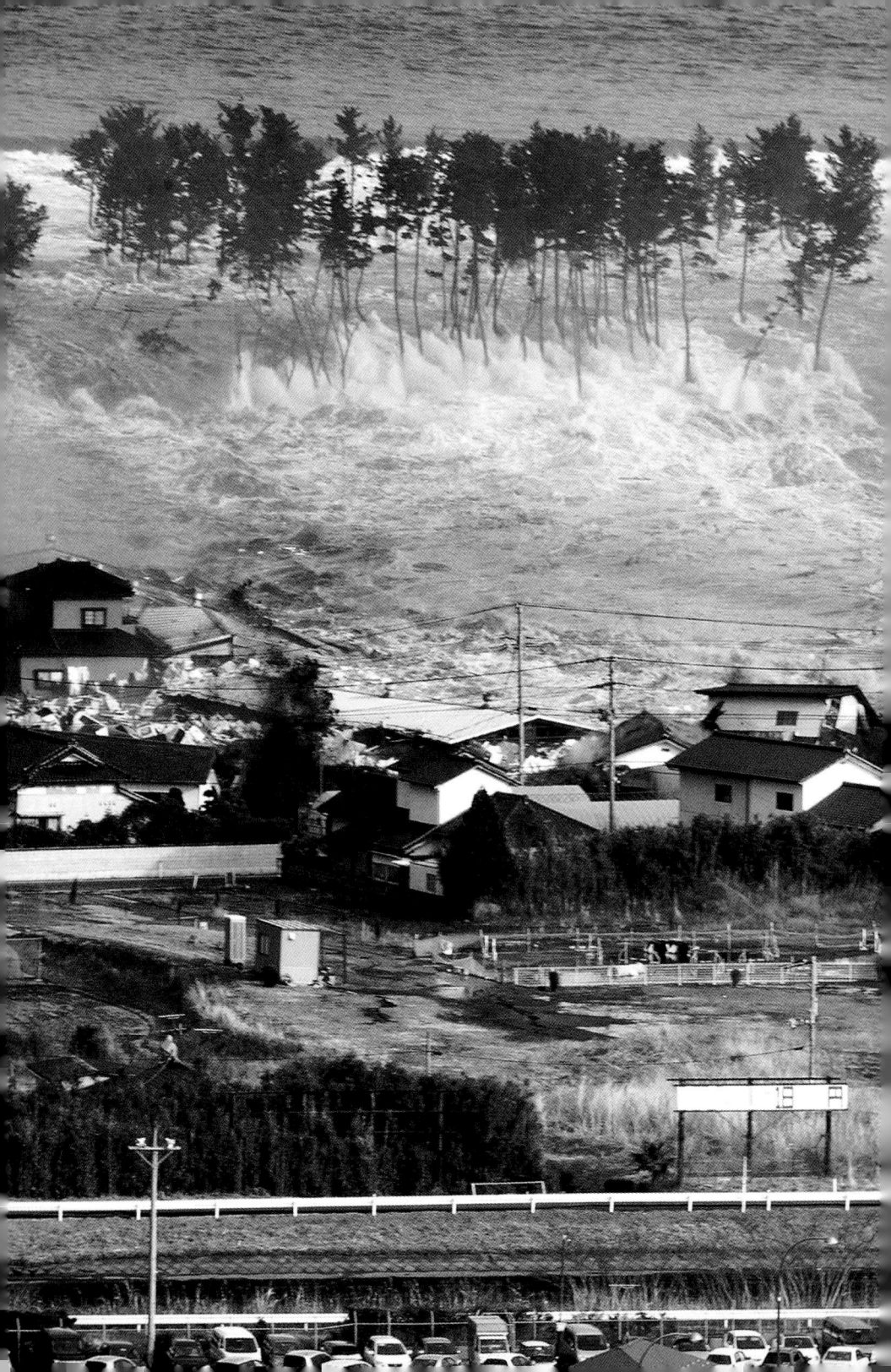

Section 4
Making the journey

Following the Tohoku earthquake, a large tsunami swallowing a group of houses at Natori city on the Pacific Ocean (see page 175). [Miyagi Prefecture, photo by Kyodo News, 11/3/2011]

The Indian transplant unit

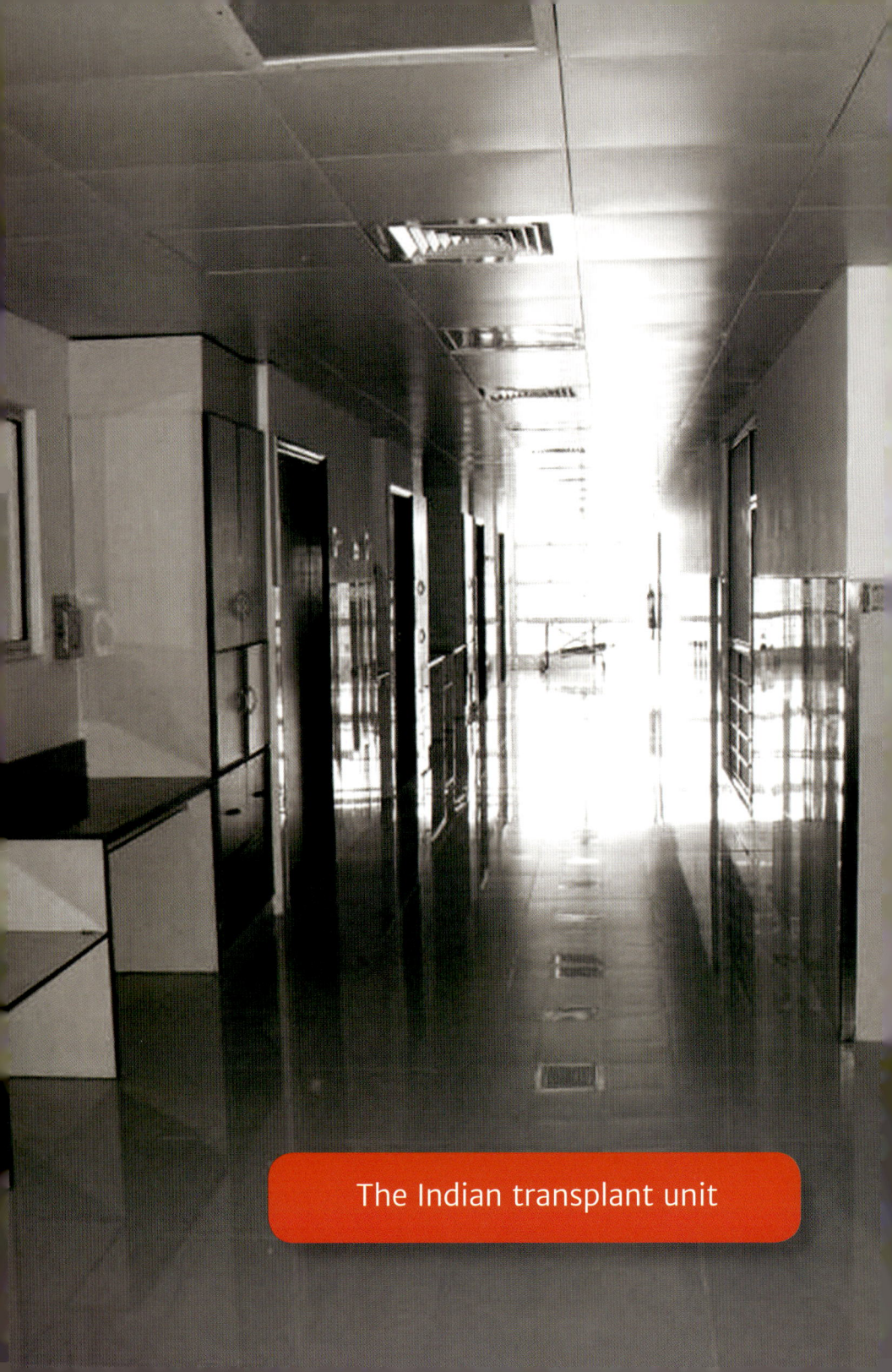

From one mother to another

Sabine Hildebrand, Head of Global Donor Recruitment, DKMS

I joined DKMS shortly after it was founded in 1991. During that time, I have had the privilege to go on courier missions around the world, bringing stem cells products to those in need. But it was in 2011, some 20 years after I had first joined DKMS, that I experienced the most precious and rewarding moment of my career.

I had been asked to deliver stem cells from a German donor to a girl in India. After a long overnight flight and overland journey, I reached the hospital, where the medical team was eagerly awaiting my arrival. After finishing all the required paperwork, I finally handed over the stem cells. The following day, I was invited to take a tour of the transplant clinic. A doctor came to pick me up and led me to another building, where I changed into sterile clothing. Upon entering the transplant clinic, I noticed a couple waiting quietly with their son in the hallway. As we got closer, the woman suddenly lowered herself to the floor. Kneeling in front of me, she began crying out loudly and gesturing hysterically.

As the dramatic scene unfolded, the doctor explained that she was the mother of the patient who was receiving the stem cells. In my eyes, I was no more than a messenger doing my job, but for the mother of the sick child, I was a hero.

As a mother of two girls, I could empathise with what she was going through, and I was overwhelmed. Despite the fact that we did not speak the same language, I took her trembling hands in mine and tried my best to comfort her. She then joined us on the tour of the clinic.

> "I felt incredibly moved and honoured to be a part of that special moment. Nothing apart from the birth of my own children has ever given me a stronger connection to life."

When we reached the end of the hallway, I saw a young patient in the last room. The face of the mother I had just befriended immediately swelled with emotion—a mixture of love, fear and hope. The patient was her daughter. I was asked, completely unexpectedly, if I wanted to observe the girl's transplant. I accepted, with the patient's consent.

It was the first time I had ever witnessed a transplant operation and it was an unforgettable experience. As the bag of stem cells continued to drip quietly, five nurses formed a circle around the girl's bed, holding each other's hands. They then prayed for the stem cells to find their way and for the treatment to be successful. I felt incredibly moved and honoured to be a part of such a special moment. Nothing apart from the birth of my own children has ever given me a stronger connection to life.

There are days when our work at DKMS seems so overwhelming. But this memory will continue to inspire me and help me stay focused on our goal, which is to delete blood cancer worldwide.

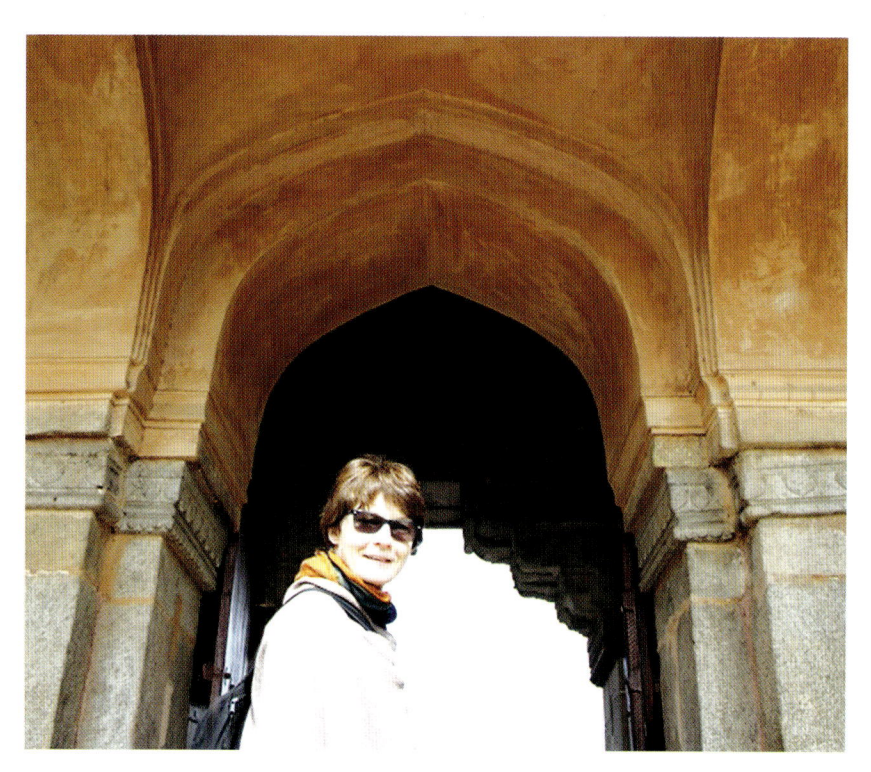

Sabine Hildebrand

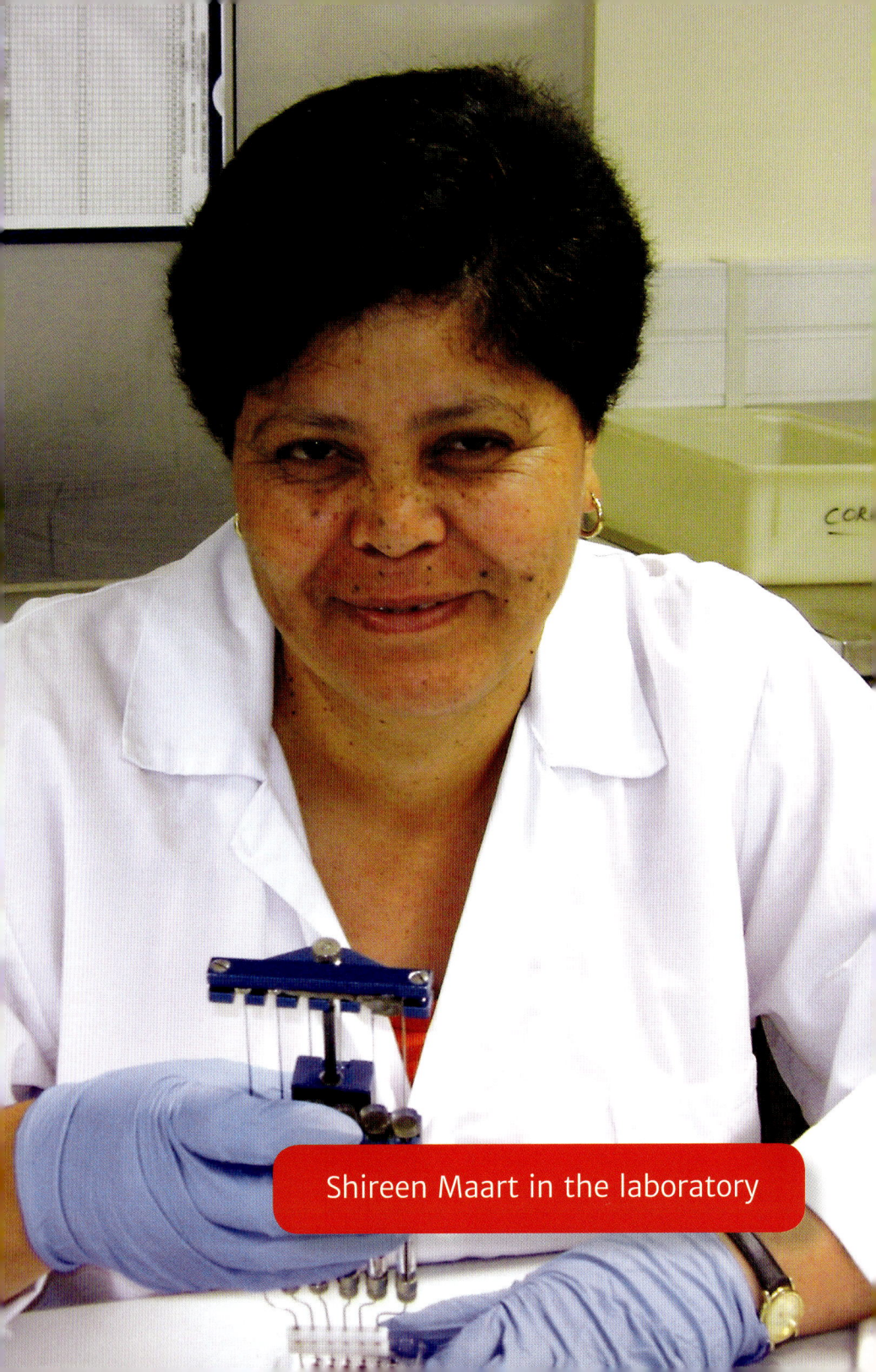

Shireen Maart in the laboratory

Last flight out of Atlanta

Shireen Maart, courier, South African Bone Marrow Registry (SABMR)

Written with the support of Terry Schlaphoff, SABMR

Despite the challenges presented by international collections—including time differences, flight connections and visas—most courier trips are uneventful. But everything does not always go according to plan.

On one occasion, I had been asked to collect stem cells from St Petersburg in Florida for a patient in Johannesburg. But shortly before my departure from the US, Hurricane Ida struck.
The hurricane caused flight delays in the southeast of the US.
My original itinerary was to fly from Tampa to Johannesburg via Atlanta, a journey of approximately 21 hours. By the time I arrived in Atlanta, I had just missed my connecting flight. My back-up plan—a flight via London—was scheduled to leave two hours later. However, there was a good chance that this other flight might also be cancelled due to the foul weather.

After many calls back and forth with my colleagues at the SABMR and our travel agent, we came up with an alternative option—a flight via Paris. This would guarantee that I could deliver the cells to the patient in time, so I did not hesitate to take the flight. And it was a good thing that I did, because Atlanta airport was closed shortly after we took off!

But that was not the end of my troubles. When I arrived in Paris, the authorities detained me because I did not have a French transit visa. Thankfully my colleagues in South Africa and I managed to convince them as to how urgent and important my case was. I was then allowed to board my flight to Johannesburg.

After travelling for more than 38 hours, I finally arrived at the hospital, just in time for the infusion of the stem cells into the patient later that day. Everyone was extremely relieved. And I personally was extremely grateful for my quick-thinking colleagues and travel agent!

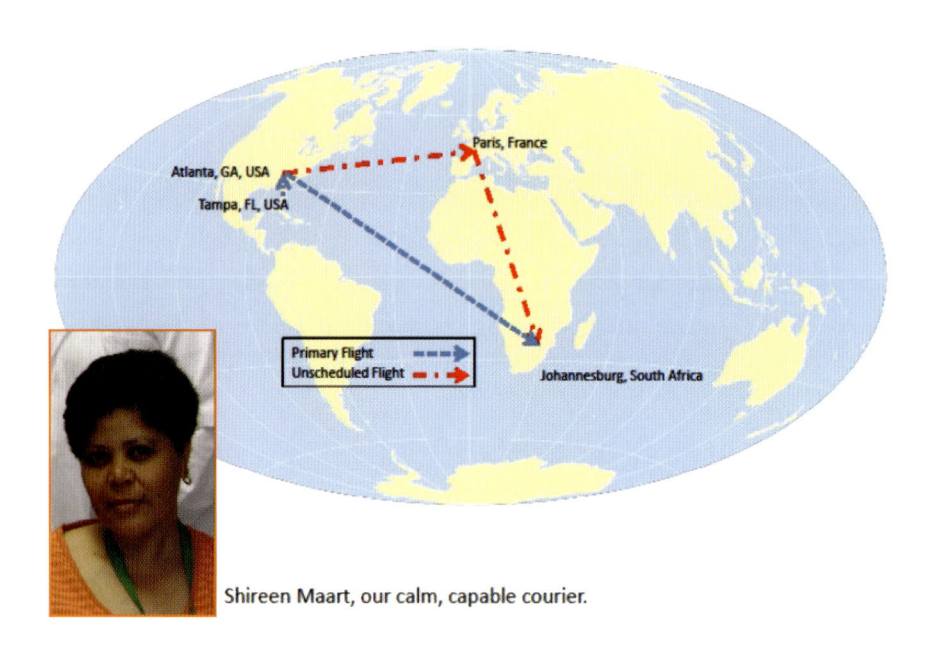

Shireen Maart, our calm, capable courier.

A number of things can pose obstacles to the international transportation of stem cells for transplant, including natural disasters, infection outbreaks, terrorism and customs issues. One of the key risks is inclement weather, which could disrupt communications and transport. Swiftly dealing with and finding solutions to these problems is crucial in order to ensure the stem cells arrive at their destination on time; it is quite literally a matter of life and death.

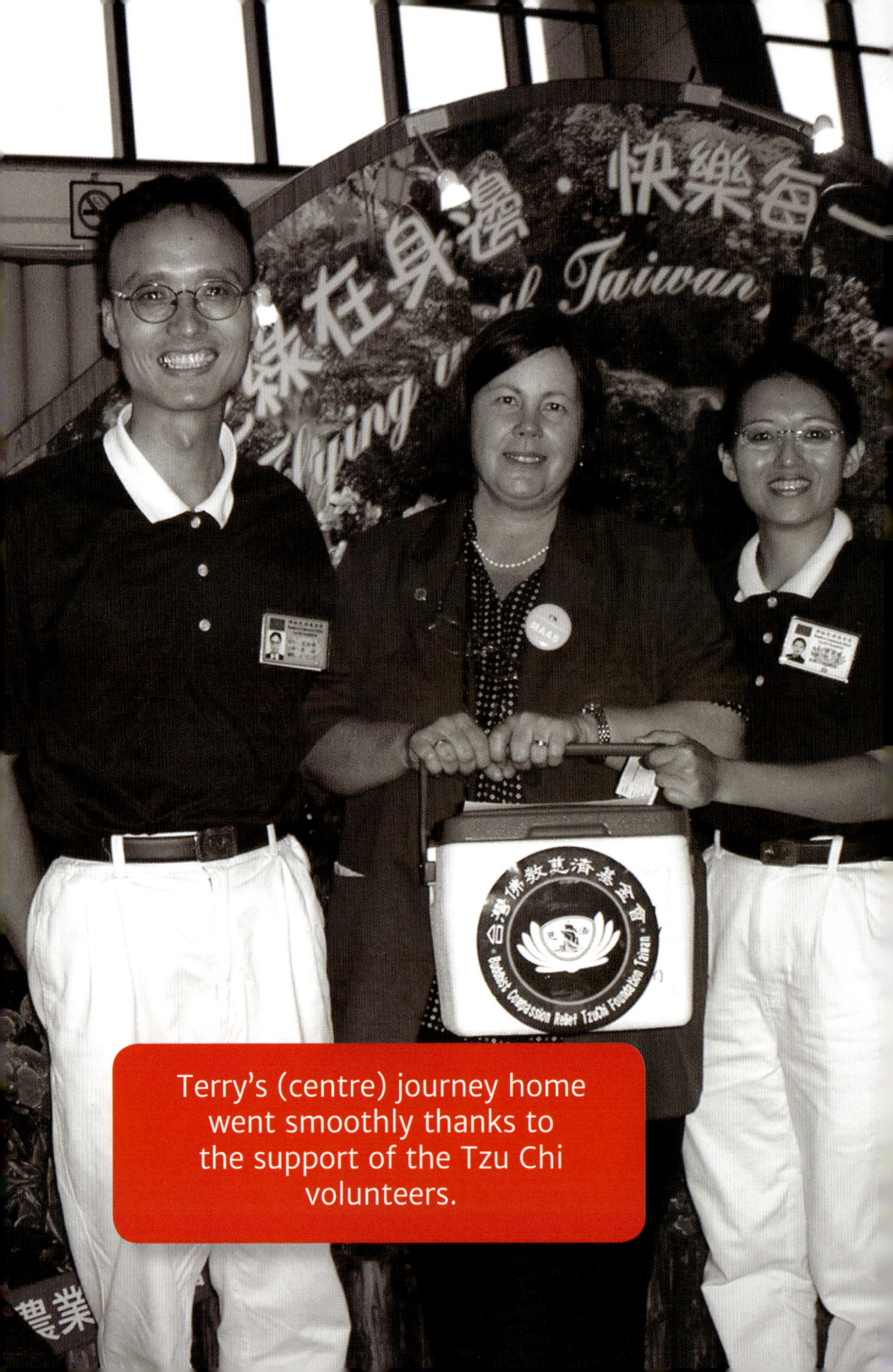

Terry's (centre) journey home went smoothly thanks to the support of the Tzu Chi volunteers.

Dealing with super typhoon Haitang

Terry Schlaphoff, South African Bone Marrow Registry (SABMR)

Stem cell couriers are trained to cope with any kind of emergency—but not many expect to have to deal with an impending typhoon! Yet this is what happened on my trip to Taiwan. It was the first time the South African Bone Marrow Registry (SABMR) had identified a suitable donor at the Buddhist Tzu Chi Stem Cell Centre, and I volunteered to make the trip to Hualien, Taiwan to collect the donor's stem cells.

The Buddhist Tzu Chi Stem Cell Centre arranged for a Buddhist nun to pick me up from the airport and send me to my hotel. On the way, the nun turned to me and uttered words that I would never forget: "Don't be afraid ... but there's a typhoon coming!"
But of course I was afraid—we do not get typhoons in South Africa! The nun explained that I would be safe inside the hotel and that the donor had already been admitted to hospital for the stem cell collection. She also said it was likely the typhoon would pass by the time the cells were collected, so it probably would not affect my departure.

Soon after I had arrived at the hotel, super typhoon Haitang made landfall with winds of more than 250km/hour. For a whole day, the hotel swayed back and forth, and I prayed. Meanwhile, the SABMR and Buddhist Tzu Chi teams got to work finding an alternative route from Taiwan to Hong Kong, from where I would head home to South Africa.

Through all of this, the donor remained in an almost deserted hospital, attended to by a very small team, to donate his valuable stem cells.

By the next day, the typhoon had passed and calm returned to Hualien. I travelled to the hospital to pick up the collected stem cells. Before my departure, Master Chen, the founder of the Buddhist Tzu Chi Stem Cell Centre, held a ceremony to bless the cells. I, too, felt very blessed that day.

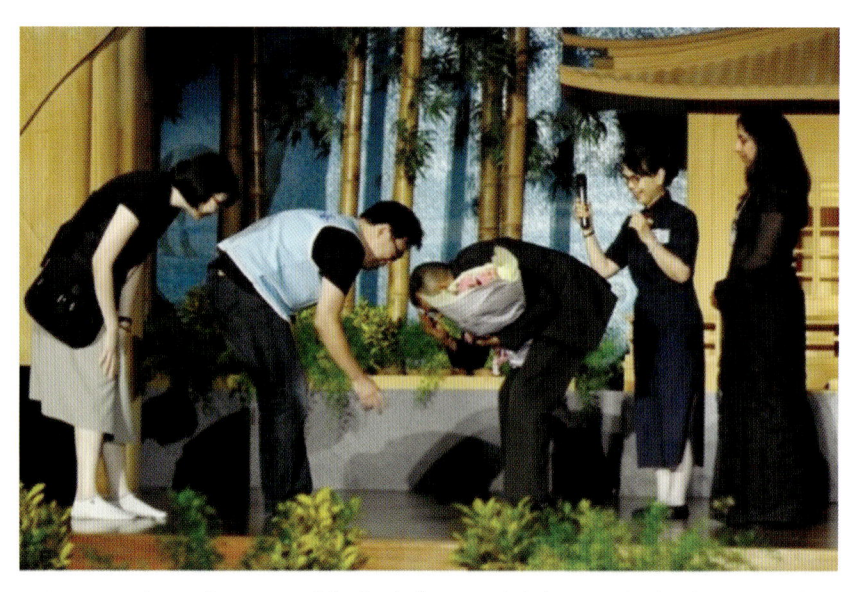

In 2013, the patient—Amrith Singh (centre right)—was invited to meet his donor in a moving ceremony held in Hualien.

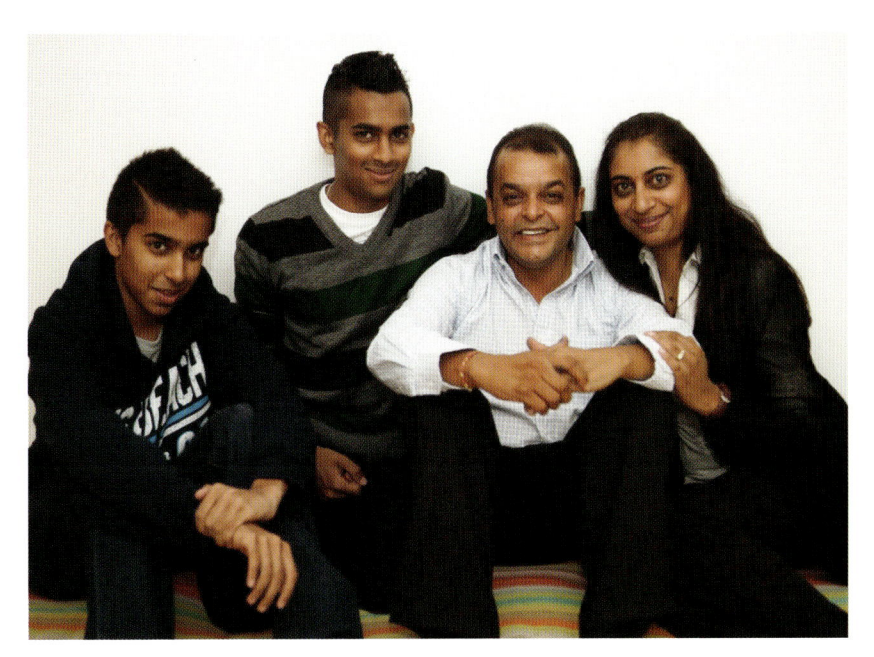

Amrith with his family

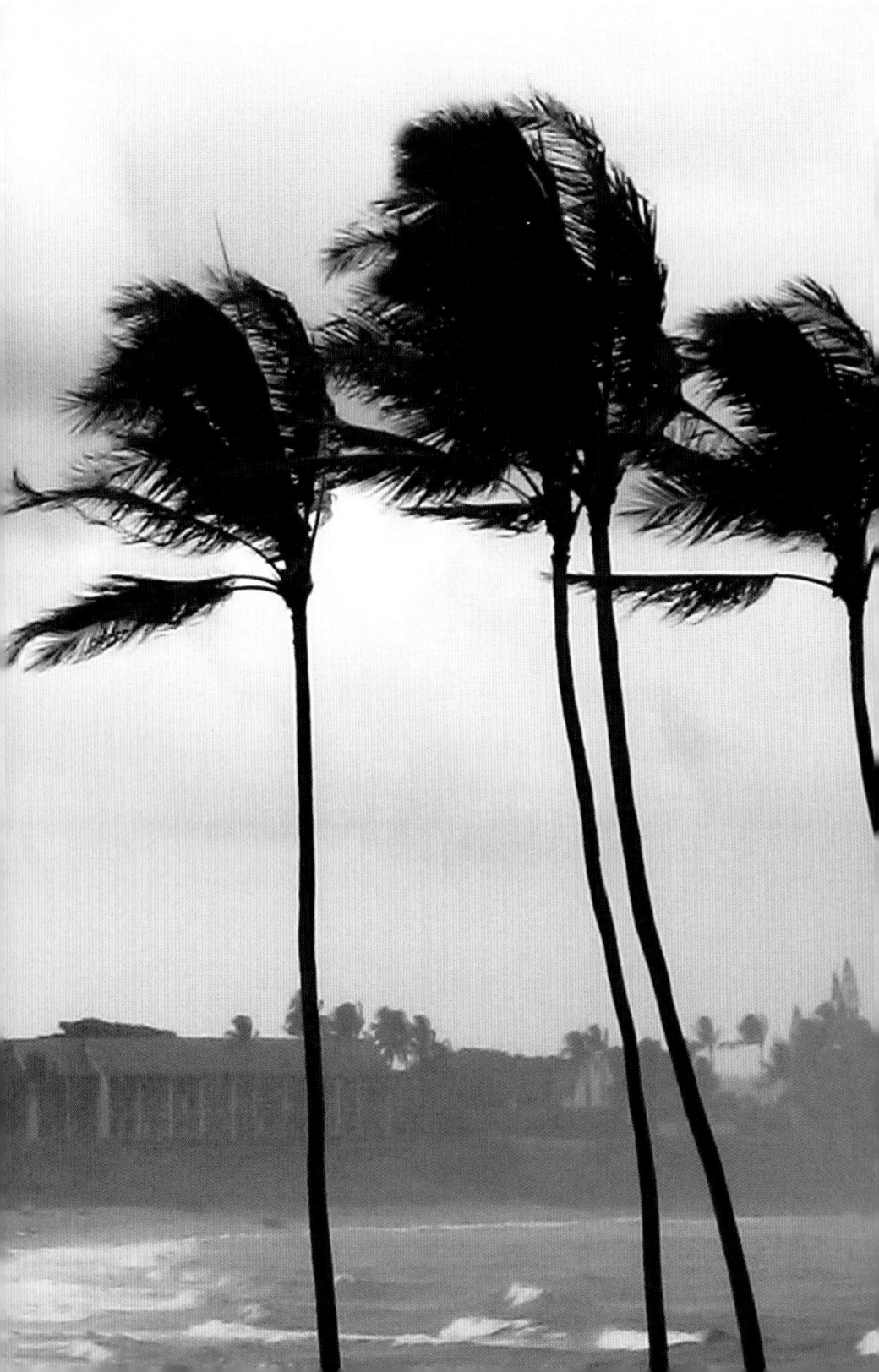

Into the eye of the storm

Peter Foster, marketing writer/editor, National Marrow Donor Program/ Be The Match

In September 2005, just weeks after Hurricane Katrina, the Gulf Coast was hit by another monstrous storm—the category 5 Hurricane Rita. Local, state and federal officials worked around the clock to send equipment and supplies to the region. Meanwhile, the Texas government ordered mandatory evacuations of the people living along the coast.

But while most of the Gulf Coast scrambled to get out of harm's way, one patient at the MD Anderson Transplant Center in Houston, Texas, had no option but to stay.

The patient urgently needed to receive the life-saving stem cells on schedule as he had already undergone preparations for a stem cell transplant. This meant that, while most people were racing to escape the city, a lone courier would have to find a way in. They would have to fly into the eye of the storm.

Back at the National Marrow Donor Program/Be The Match Coordinating Center in Minneapolis, Minnesota, an emergency response team was already in action, preparing for different scenarios and arranging extra support for patients, donors and couriers.

Every courier needs to be resourceful, flexible and a creative problem-solver. But getting the stem cells into Houston would be especially challenging. Not only would the courier have to find transportation, they would also most likely have to ride out the hurricane once they were there.

We identified Mary Minke Lappegaard as the best person for the job. Mary had extensive experience as a professional logistics coordinator for the National Marrow Donor Program/Be The Match. She also had a realistic understanding of the difficulties she would face and the personal resolve required to overcome these challenges.

> "...her role as a courier was successfully fulfilled. But what she did not know was that the real adventure was only just beginning."

Armed with the documents that identified her as a courier and gave her priority travel clearance, Mary set off on her journey. After collecting the stem cells, she flew to Atlanta, Georgia, where flights were already being cancelled due to the bad weather. Boarding a small plane, she braced herself for what was certain to be a bumpy ride.

All roads to Houston International Airport were closed, so Mary flew to Houston's second major airport, around 45 miles from her destination, where she was greeted by a police escort.

And it was just as well—there were no taxis or rental cars available, and local and state officials had ordered mandatory evacuations. Around 1.5 million Texans were using all lanes in both directions to exit the region. Mary and her travel companions found themselves driving along the hard shoulder, cautiously making their way into the city against the stream of oncoming traffic.

When Mary finally arrived at the hospital and delivered the critical stem cells in time for the transplant, her role as a courier was successfully fulfilled. But what she did not know was that the real adventure was only just beginning.

Back at the hotel where she was staying, tensions were rising. Many evacuees had already made the hotel their temporary home after Hurricane Katrina. Traumatised and disoriented, some were nearing a state of panic now that another hurricane was approaching. Hotel staff did their best to provide whatever reassurances they could. They called people together, advised them to close windows and curtains, and to fill their bathtubs with water—both for emergency drinking water, and in the hope that the extra weight would help stabilise the building.

As the storm intensified, many people moved their mattresses out of their rooms and into the hallways to get away from the windows.

At that point, even moving through the hallways was a daunting proposition; one had to step over and around groups of people huddled together—whole families with small children and older people who had been displaced from their homes. Some had already lost neighbours, friends or family members, and did not even know if they had homes to return to.

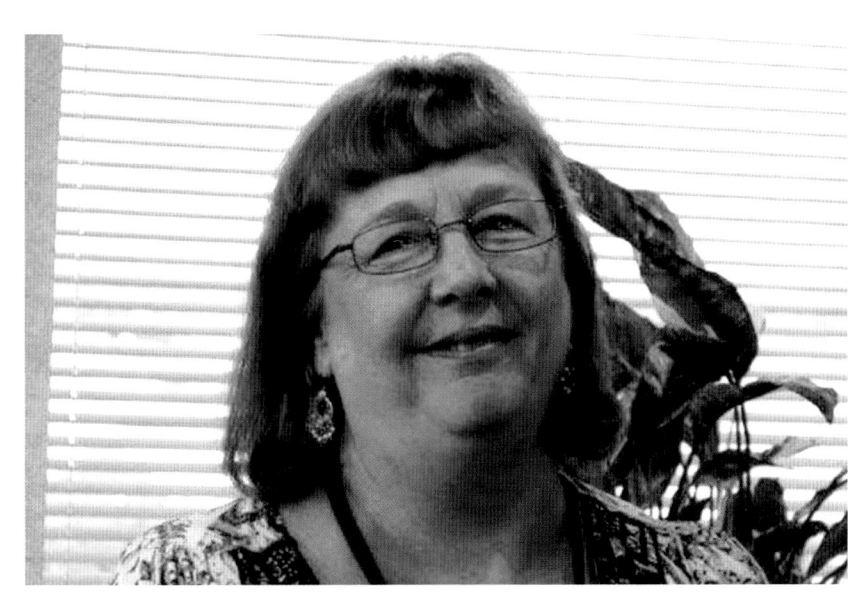

Mary Lappegaard who braved hurricane **Katrina**.

Into the eye of the storm

Mary watched the storm unfold through her hotel window, which was criss-crossed with tape to minimise the threat of flying glass. Although it flexed ominously in the howling wind, the window held secure. Mary looked on in awe as street signs fluttered, bent and twisted under the assault. Steel newspaper boxes, ripped from their moorings, tumbled and crashed down the street.

> The 2005 Atlantic hurricane season brought with it a series of major tropical cyclones that caused over $150 billion in damages and left thousands dead. Hurricane Katrina was the most destructive, while Hurricane Rita was the most intense ever observed in the Gulf of Mexico. Land, air and sea transport was significantly affected during this time of crisis.

Hurricane Rita came ashore at around 3.30am that night, with winds that reached 120 mph. It knocked out power for more than one million people, sparked multiple fires, and swamped Louisiana shoreline towns with a 15-foot storm surge.

By morning, the worst of the storm had passed—but the ordeal was far from over. For the next five days, Mary was confined to the hotel. There was no power, no air conditioning and little more to eat and drink than the stale rolls, leftover butter and remaining bottled water that the staff doled out. Mary was free to leave her room, but there was nowhere to go. There were no businesses or relief centres nearby that could offer better conditions.

Through it all, Mary kept in contact with the team at the coordinating centre, who provided updates and called her parents to let them know they were doing everything in their power to bring Mary home. Several days later, the emergency response team was finally able to arrange for a private car to pick her up.

After the storm, Mary was one of 18 people the National Marrow Donor Program/Be The Match specially commended for their selfless actions during the hurricane. Besides couriers, these people included donors, emergency coordinators, police officers and others who overcame every obstacle to help a patient in need. The commitment shown by these individuals demonstrates the global transplant community's exemplary dedication to saving lives.

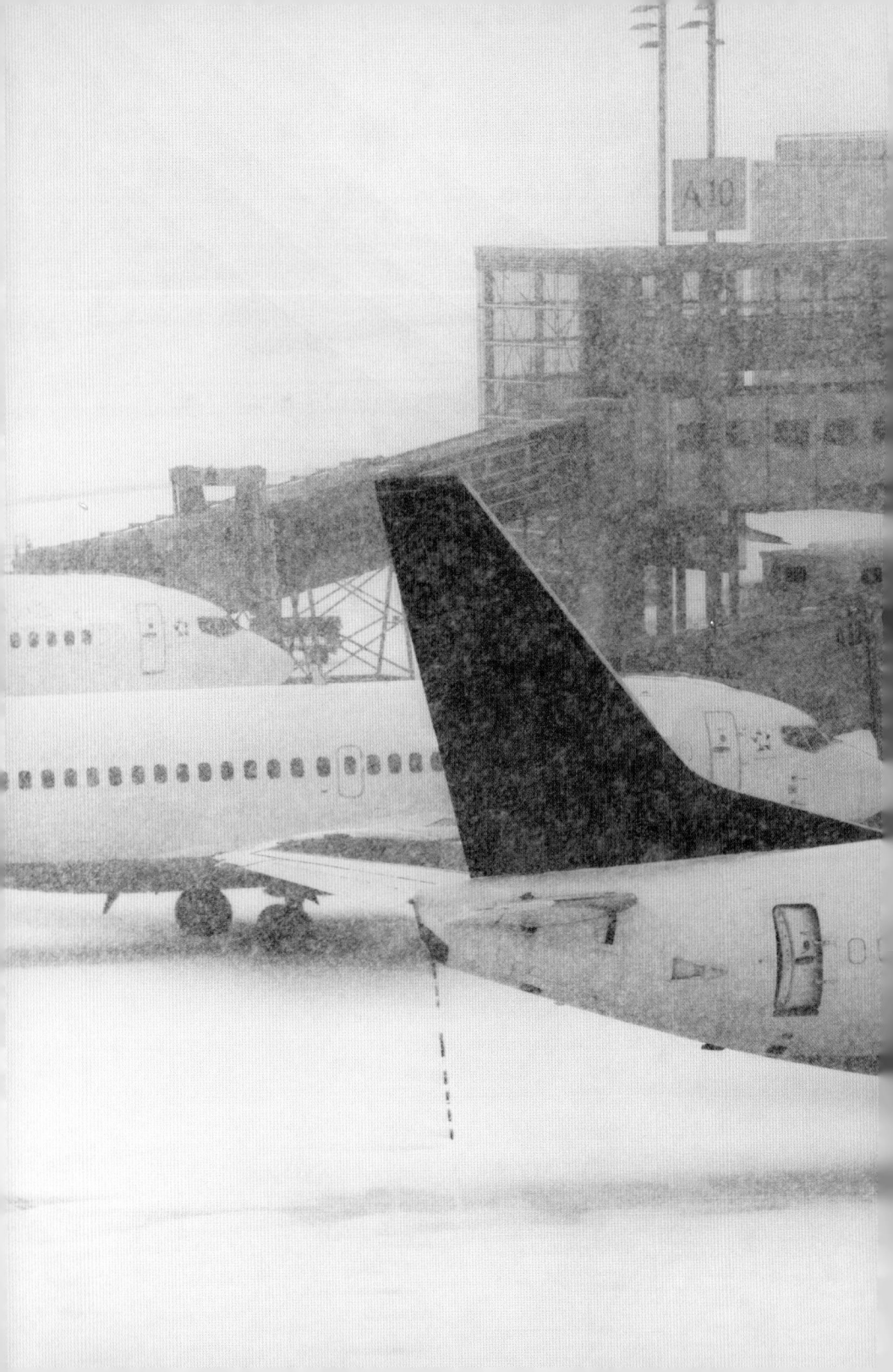

Planes, trains and automobiles

Peter Foster, marketing writer/editor, National Marrow Donor Program/ Be The Match

In the John Hughes film 'Planes, Trains and Automobiles', characters played by Steve Martin and John Candy face a series of obstacles as they struggle to get from New York to Chicago on time for Thanksgiving. Watching them become increasingly anxious and frustrated as they were repeatedly stalled, blocked and rerouted makes for a great comedy. But when bone marrow courier Tiffany Preston experienced this dilemma, it was anything but a laughing matter—because the life of a patient depended on her making this journey successfully.

As an HLA specialist at Inland Northwest Blood Center in Spokane, Washington—a centre affiliated with the National Marrow Donor Program/Be The Match—Tiffany was an experienced courier. On any other day, the relatively short 280-mile trip from Spokane to Seattle might have seemed little more than an errand. After all, it was only a 45-minute flight.

But the day Tiffany was scheduled to depart was no ordinary day, with a winter storm dumping a record-breaking 17 inches of snow at Spokane International Airport in a 24-hour period. The city had declared a snow emergency, which meant that every available ploughing crew was being deployed 24/7 to clear roads. Schools and government offices were closed. Garbage pick-up was suspended. Buses were cancelled. And police urged people to stay at home.

For Tiffany, however, staying home was not an option. A patient waiting for a stem cell transplant in Seattle urgently needed the donor cells she was carrying. Once the conditioning regimen had destroyed the patient's diseased marrow, effectively wiping out their blood and immune system, it was crucial that the healthy cells be infused as soon as possible. Tiffany had to get to the hospital in Seattle; the patient's life depended on it.

One of Tiffany's co-workers, Roxann, volunteered to drive the six miles to the airport in her four-wheel-drive vehicle. They powered through the ice and snow, passing a number of collisions and stranded cars on the side of the road. Finally, they reached Spokane International Airport. It was no surprise that Tiffany's original flight had been cancelled. She pulled out documents explaining that she was carrying life-saving cells and requested special status, which, if accepted by the airline, would give her priority departure on the first available flight. But by then the snow was falling so fast that ploughs could not keep the runways clear, and the planes could not be loaded or de-iced quickly enough.

> "As the day wore on, flight after flight was cancelled. It soon became clear that another mode of transportation was needed."

As the day wore on, flight after flight was cancelled. It soon became clear that another mode of transportation was needed. Roxann offered to try driving Tiffany all the way to Seattle, but the transplant centre requested that, for everyone's safety, no one should attempt to drive in those conditions. Instead, they asked Tiffany to keep hold of the product overnight and try to catch a flight in the morning. But come morning, conditions still had not improved.

With flying no longer an option, it was time to put plan B into action: the train. But trains were also significantly delayed. It was 3.30pm by the time Tiffany was finally able to board a train for Seattle. Just two hours later, the train ground to a halt in

Wenatchee, east of the Cascade Mountain Range. Another train had broken down up ahead and there was no guessing when it might be cleared.

Back to plan A. Tiffany boarded a plane heading from Wenatchee to Seattle—but once again it was not to be. The seal on the plane door was frozen and would not shut properly. Several attempts to heat, de-ice and reseal the door resulted in Tiffany and the other passengers having to disembark and reboard multiple times. Just before midnight, Tiffany exited the airplane for the last time. The flight was a no-go.

> More than 55 unrelated donor stem cell transplants are performed every day around the world. Of these, 25 are couriered across borders from the donor's location to the recipient, who could be based in a completely different part of the world.

Fortunately, during that time, the emergency response team in Minneapolis had contacted Washington State Highway Patrol. It was agreed that they would coordinate rides, transferring Tiffany from one highway patrol SUV to another as they transported her across three districts. It was a little past midnight before Tiffany was back on the road again.

At around 2am, Tiffany confirmed that the weather was starting to clear and that they were making good progress. And at 3.30am, the team finally got the news they had been waiting to hear—a simple message that read 'Product delivered'.

This story demonstrates that delivering life-saving stem cells safely and on time, no matter what, requires tremendous dedication, determination and quick thinking—from both volunteer couriers and the entire transplant community who supports them. Everyone involved is 100 per cent committed to doing everything they can to help a patient get the transplant they need.

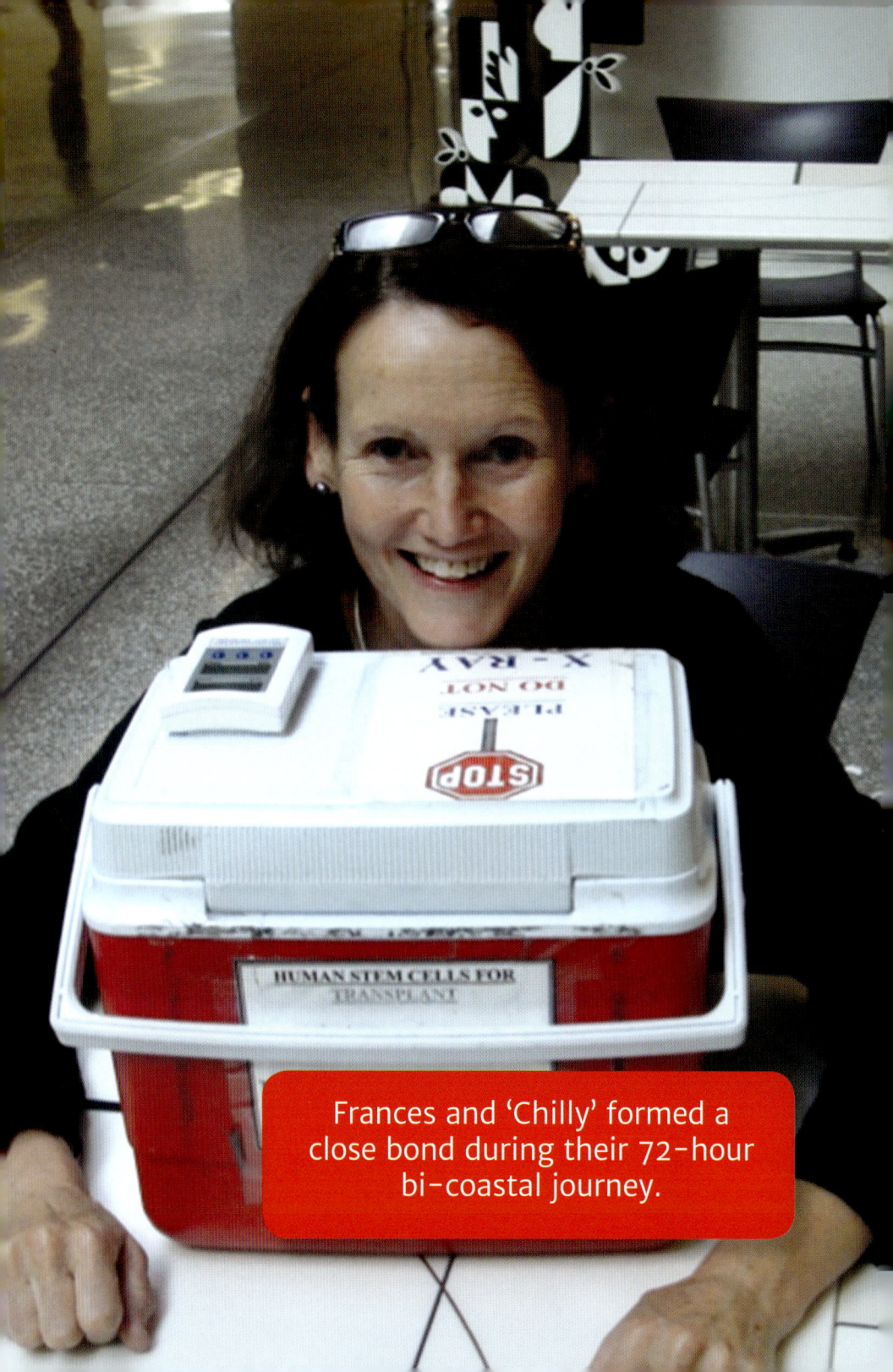

Frances and 'Chilly' formed a close bond during their 72-hour bi-coastal journey.

From Washington DC to Wellington NZ in 72 hours

Frances Fitzjohn, New Zealand Blood Donor Registry

Stem cells ... check.
Chilly bin ... check.
Flight tickets ... check.
Patient ready and waiting for transplant ... check.

I was ready to transport my precious cargo of stem cells to my waiting patient. Now all that was needed was for a little snowstorm to be added to the mix!

Having made it to Washington DC on what turned out to be the last flight into Dulles International Airport before the snowstorm started, the question was: how on earth would I be able to get out of this snowy city with the stem cells that the patient was waiting for? I still had two days before my flight was due to leave, and anything could happen during that time. And it did; even more snow fell!

Luckily, I had the amazing team at the New Zealand Bone Marrow Donor Registry behind me. They swung into action and worked through our options together with our travel agents and our colleagues in the US. A final game plan was worked out and it sounded promising. The stem cells and I would take a train to New York, and then head home to Wellington via San Francisco.

After enjoying two days of slippery sightseeing in DC, I made my way to the collection centre by taxi to pick up the stem cells. From there I was bundled into another taxi along with my chilly bin full of stem cells ('Chilly' for short). But when we got to the station, it seemed as if most of DC was trying to get onto the same train as me!

I explained my situation to the staff and, before I had a chance to panic, someone raced me through some 'No entry' doors and threw Chilly and me onto a train bound for New York. By 6pm that evening, we found ourselves on a busy NYC street. After checking in at our hotel, Chilly and I went down to dinner. I arranged for the ice packs to be stored in a freezer overnight, as they still had a long way to travel.

> "And I was pleased to see that they were given pride of place among the frozen margaritas and piña coladas in the cocktail bar's freezer!"

And I was pleased to see that they were given pride of place among the frozen margaritas and piña coladas in the cocktail bar's freezer! I woke up the next day feeling fresh and ready to fly to San Francisco, so I went down to the lobby early to check out. I was again greeted by crowds of people. What did the other guests know that I didn't? I soon found out—JFK airport was closed. Looking outside, I could see why—the snow had followed us and was now causing chaos here too.

I decided to head to the airport anyway. But when I finally got to JFK, it was like a ghost town. I had my choice of seating areas, full run of the food/drink machines and extremely limited conversation! But Chilly and I were just happy to be first on the scene. Hopefully this would put us at the front of the queue if any flights were able to take off.

Later in the afternoon, after a slight reprieve in the weather, a couple of smaller planes took off and I heard that there might be a flight to San Francisco leaving soon. Finally my patience was rewarded and I was handed a prized boarding pass.

Our plane was towed into its bay and de-iced. Eventually, we were directed to the gate and then boarded. The plane was de-iced again and everything looked promising. But by the time it was ready to taxi off, it had to be de-iced another time. Surely it had to be third time lucky? I was right. Finally, Chilly and I were on our way to snow-free San Francisco.

I felt an immense sense of relief when we finally boarded our Air New Zealand flight to Auckland. The crew was great and had dry ice all ready and waiting for us. My ice packs had not really had a chance to melt, but with hours to go, I needed to make sure that the stem cells stayed at the correct temperature all the way home.

Because we arrived late into Auckland, we had to make an overnight stop before flying on to Wellington. Early the next morning, we were finally winging our way to our final destination and to the lovely man who had been waiting patiently for his cells for 72 hours. What a journey!

> A courier's job is fulfilling, exciting and challenging. While most trips are uneventful, almost anything can and has happened during their journeys as they seek to deliver their life-saving cargo safely. The basic requirements of a stem cell courier can be summarised with four Rs: responsible, resourceful, resilient and 'ready for anything'.

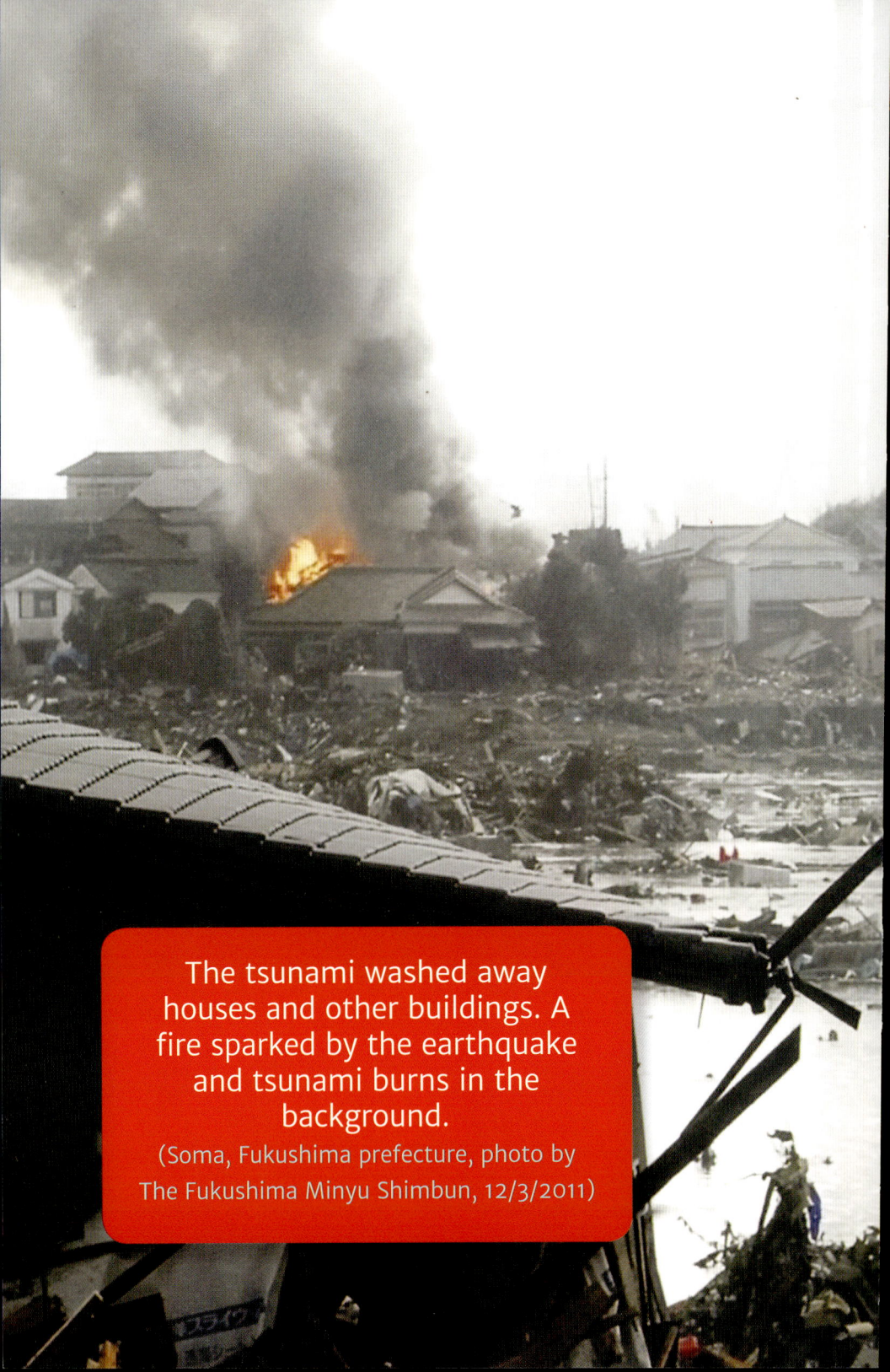

The tsunami washed away houses and other buildings. A fire sparked by the earthquake and tsunami burns in the background.
(Soma, Fukushima prefecture, photo by The Fukushima Minyu Shimbun, 12/3/2011)

Great East Japan earthquake

Azusa Sato, Japan Marrow Donor Program

On 11 March 2011, a record 9.0 magnitude earthquake struck off the Pacific coast of Tōhoku, Japan. It caused a huge tsunami with waves more than 10 metres high. One hour later, this tsunami caused the cooling system at Fukushima Daiichi Nuclear Power Plant to fail, resulting in a nuclear meltdown and the release of radioactive materials into the surrounding environment.

Immediately after the disaster, our main priorities were to confirm the safety of both our donors and coordinators, and to assess the damages to the transplant and collection centres around the disaster zone.

While we were able to verify that all our donors and coordinators were safe, they sadly did not escape personal tragedies. Many lost their family members during the tsunami. For some, the buildings of companies they worked for were destroyed, so they lost their jobs. And those with homes within the nuclear evacuation area had to be relocated to temporary lodgings.

Because telephone and mobile networks were down, we reverted to communicating with donors by posting on notice boards at our centres. One week after the disaster, our centres in Tokyo began collecting and sending bone marrow to patients in affected areas. Three months later, our transplant centres in the Tōhoku area were also able to resume full operation.

Our coordinators have since said how much they admire the dedication of our donors and their families in the aftermath of the disaster, and their willingness to help others despite their own misfortunes. Through this experience, we have deepened and strengthened our ability to work as a team and to manage future crises.

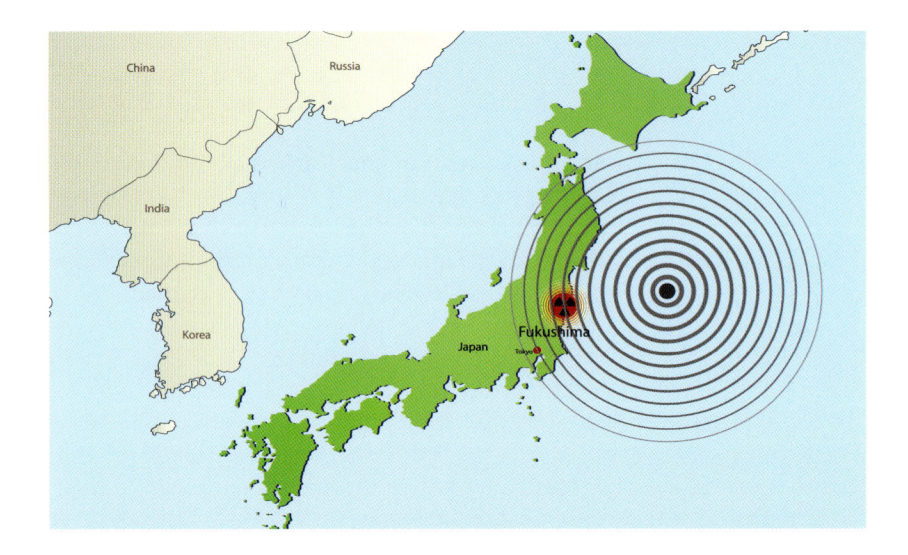

For instance, we have created a donor correspondence manual for use in emergency situations such as earthquakes. And we now see the value in using donor centres for distributing information. We hope that what we have learnt will help other organisations that may unfortunately find themselves in similar situations in the future.

> "After losing people I knew to the tsunami, I understand a little about the feelings of patients who are in need of a transplant. So how could I refuse to help?"
>
> Anonymous Japanese donor

The 2011 Tōhoku earthquake which caused a tsunami, and the subsequent nuclear meltdown at the Fukushima power plant, was a disaster that affected many lives. Communications and transport channels were also severely disrupted. The response of the Japanese people was systematic, disciplined and compassionate. This includes the exemplary response of the haematopoietic stem cell transplant community in Japan, which responded in full force to contain the issue and support the many patients who were waiting for a transplant.

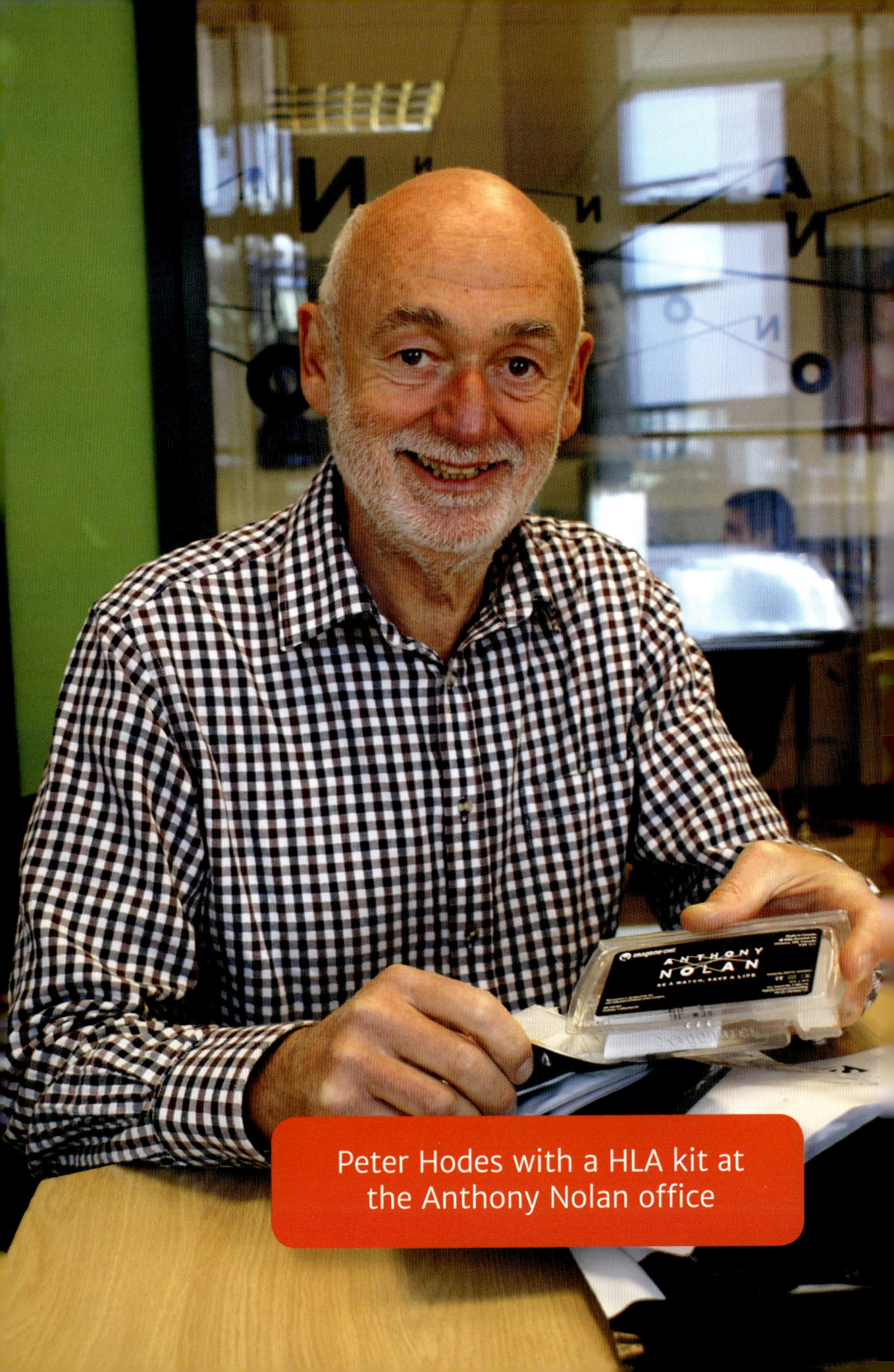

Peter Hodes with a HLA kit at the Anthony Nolan office

Keep calm and courier on

Peter Hodes, an Anthony Nolan volunteer courier living in London, UK

Written with the support of Jo Badger and Emma Radway-Bright at Anthony Nolan

I have done more than 50 pick-ups since starting as a courier in March 2012. Because I am self-employed, I'm able to fit in the trips around my working, social, cultural and charitable life. It is a wonderful mix. Sometimes I feel that my feet don't touch the ground, and that's just how I like it.

The furthest I have travelled is to Brisbane in Australia. The return journey to Royal Manchester Children's Hospital took 37 hours in total. It included two flights, a long layover in Kuala Lumpur and then a train to Manchester, but the sense of satisfaction I experienced when I handed over the stem cells, particularly as they were for a child, was immense. I slept very well that night!

I have also had to overcome tremendous hurdles to get stem cells back on time. In June 2013, I picked up stem cells in Providence, Rhode Island, and was bringing them back to the UK for a patient. When I arrived at the airport with my precious cargo, I discovered that the first hurricane of the season was working its way up the eastern seaboard of the US. My flight to Washington DC was so delayed that I would miss my onward connection to London. I explained the seriousness of the situation to the check-in clerk.

She immediately dropped everything, told her colleague to continue checking in other passengers and then proceeded to bust a gut to get me back to London.

After numerous phone calls, lots of tapping on her computer keyboard and a flight being held on the ground for twenty minutes, I was rerouted via Newark. Needless to say that when I boarded the plane—a tiny propeller one—the passengers were none too pleased. Then there was the problem of finding space for my box, as the overhead lockers were too small and it wouldn't fit under my seat. It ended up in the cockpit between the pilot and co-pilot!

> "Amazingly, I arrived at my final destination in Oxford two-and-a-half hours earlier than expected—much to the delight of the staff there!"

We landed in Newark in a downpour, the result of the approaching tropical storm, with just enough time for me to board the plane to London. Amazingly, I arrived at my final destination in Oxford two-and-a-half hours earlier than expected—much to the delight of the staff there!

I get a huge sense of satisfaction from being an Anthony Nolan courier. Every time I deliver a bag of stem cells, I know that I am helping to potentially save a life. It is a remarkable charity and I hope that it will have a role for me for many years to come.

> Anthony Nolan provides training for volunteer couriers covering all aspects of the work involved in transporting stem cells safely and effectively. The couriers must also attend additional training sessions twice a year to ensure their skills and knowledge stay up-to-date. Volunteers are initially asked to make three trips to transplant centres in Greater London, followed by a further three around the UK, before they are considered for international journeys.

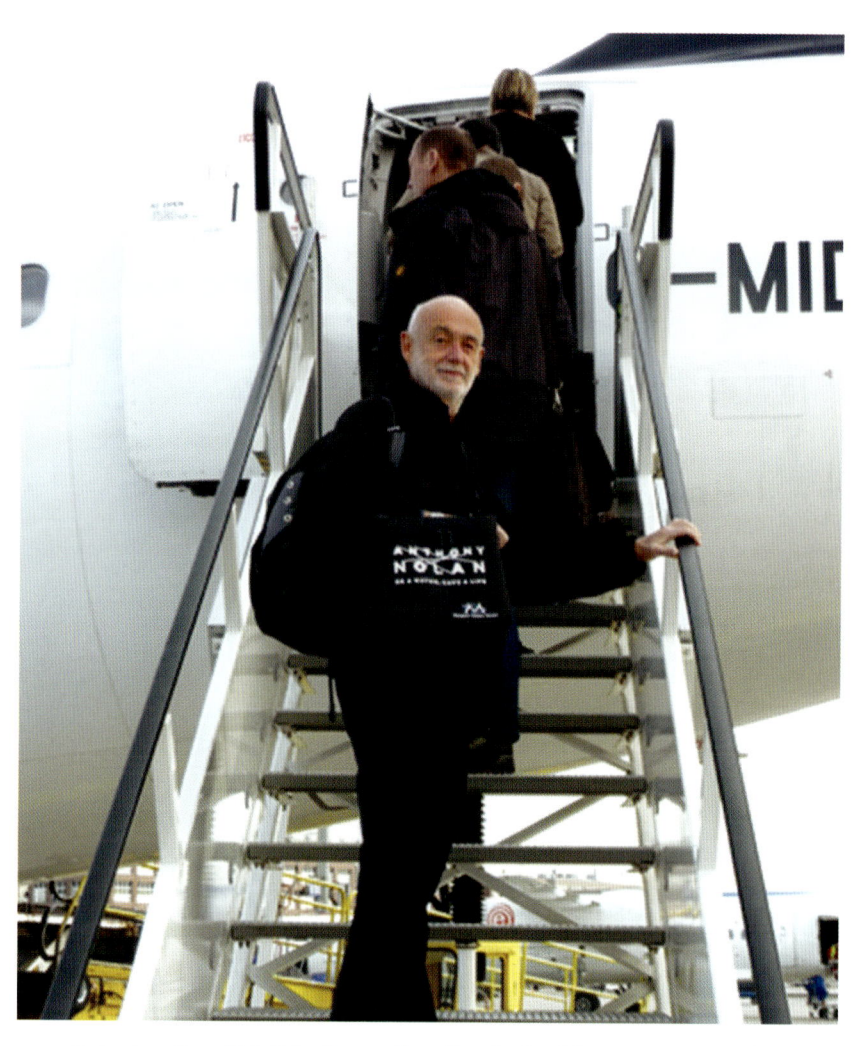

Peter has faced his fair share of hurdles during his years as a courier.

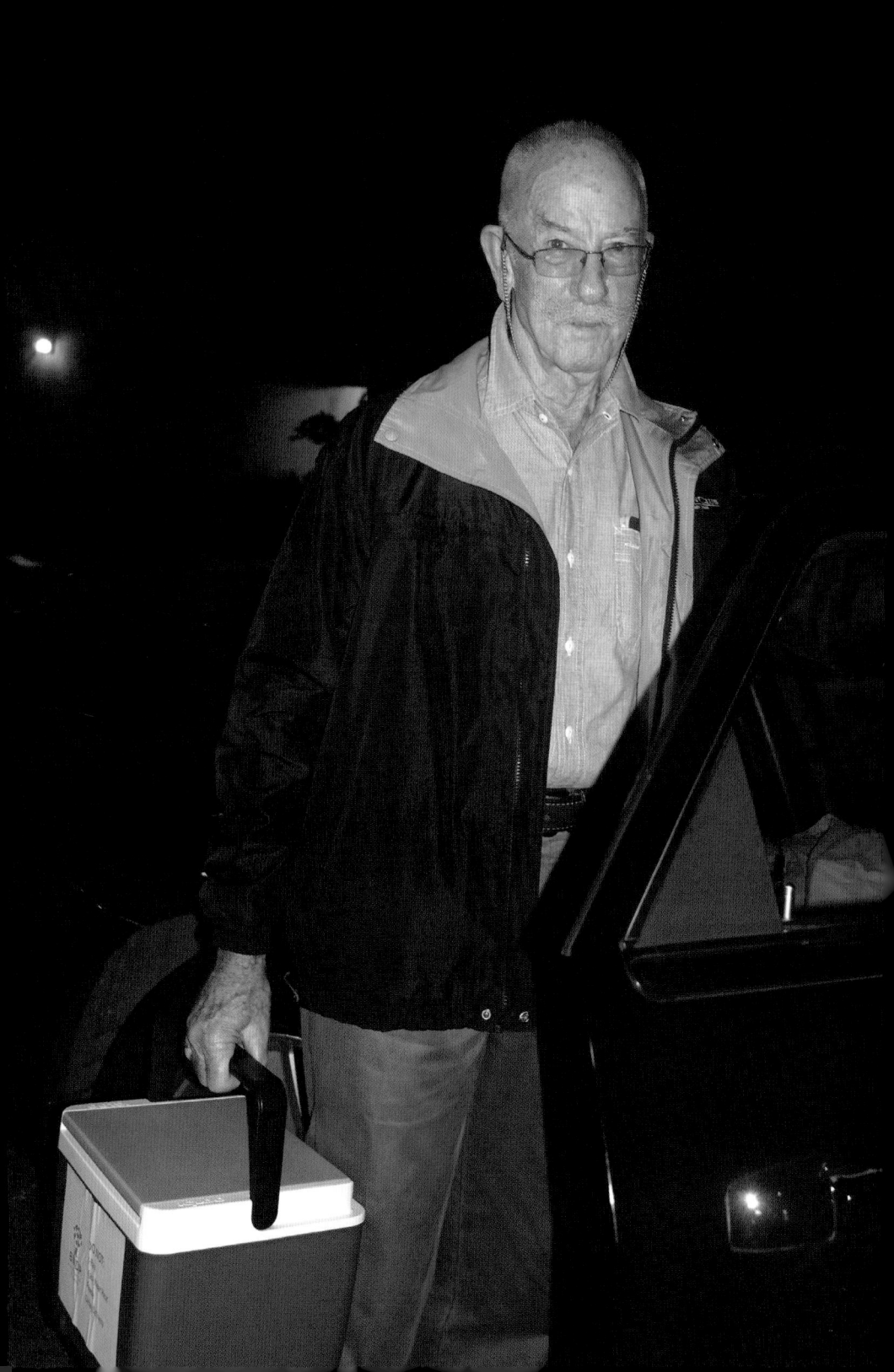

Stepping up

Roger Prior, volunteer courier for the Singapore Bone Marrow Donor Programme (BMDP)

My involvement with the Singapore Bone Marrow Donor Programme (BMDP) began in 1996 when our eldest son needed a transplant. It was a very new registry at that time and was mainly set up to meet the needs of the local population, which is Chinese, Indian and Malay. So while we did not find a matching donor locally, the registry played a vital role in leading the global search and remains very important to me.

When the BMDP needed support setting up an international courier programme, I felt that it was a very tangible way in which I could help. I was already an experienced traveller and all the problems of immigration, security and flight delays were nothing new to me. I have since flown more than 100 trips—usually bringing the product back to Singapore, but sometimes delivering to neighbouring Malaysia or Thailand. I have collected products from all over the world, including the US, Canada, the UK, Germany, Japan, Hong Kong and Taiwan. It was also my task to collect our first-ever procurement from China.

There are many highlights to this role, and working together with Singapore Airlines is one of them. Although we are economy-class passengers paying the lowest fare, we always get VIP treatment from them, and their staff go above and beyond to help us out. In return, we usually give them a teddy bear or some other small souvenir to say thank you!

One trip with Singapore Airlines that especially stands out is when I was bringing a product back from Houston in the US. We pushed back from the air bridge for an on-time departure but, as we were queuing to take off, a severe electrical storm struck. The control tower was hit by lightning a number of times and knocked out of action, and the airport was closed until they could find a temporary control tower. We eventually departed three hours late, only to receive an on-board announcement that severe head winds would delay us even further.

> "The captain notified Singapore Airlines and then stepped on the gas so that we landed slightly earlier than had been originally announced."

The flight was now due to land in San Francisco a matter of minutes after my connecting flight to Singapore was scheduled to take off. Although I was not optimistic they could do anything about it, I told one of the cabin crew that I was carrying some bone marrow bound for a patient in Singapore, and asked if she could inform the captain. The response I received was fantastic. The captain notified Singapore Airlines and then stepped on the gas so that we landed slightly earlier than had been originally announced. As the doors opened, I was delivered into the arms of a Singapore Airlines representative.

With 400 passengers already strapped in and ready to leave for Singapore, we raced across the terminal to join them. I was pushed on board, the door was slammed shut behind me and we were pushing back from the terminal even before I had buckled up.

The product was delivered on time and, as so many times before on much less dramatic trips, this was thanks to the huge number of people who came together in support of our work. While not everyone can be a donor, in my travels through different airports and countries I have met many individuals who have stepped up and played their own part in our mission to save lives.

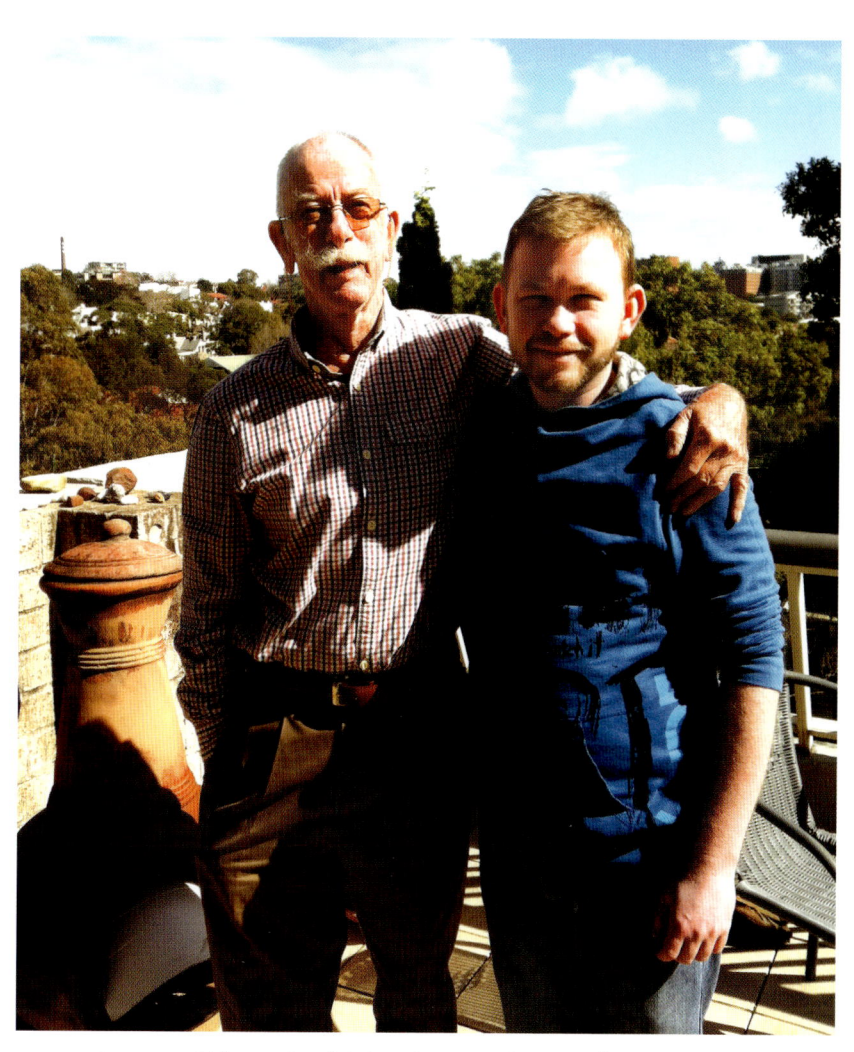

Roger and his son Daniel (see Page 40 for story "No big deal").

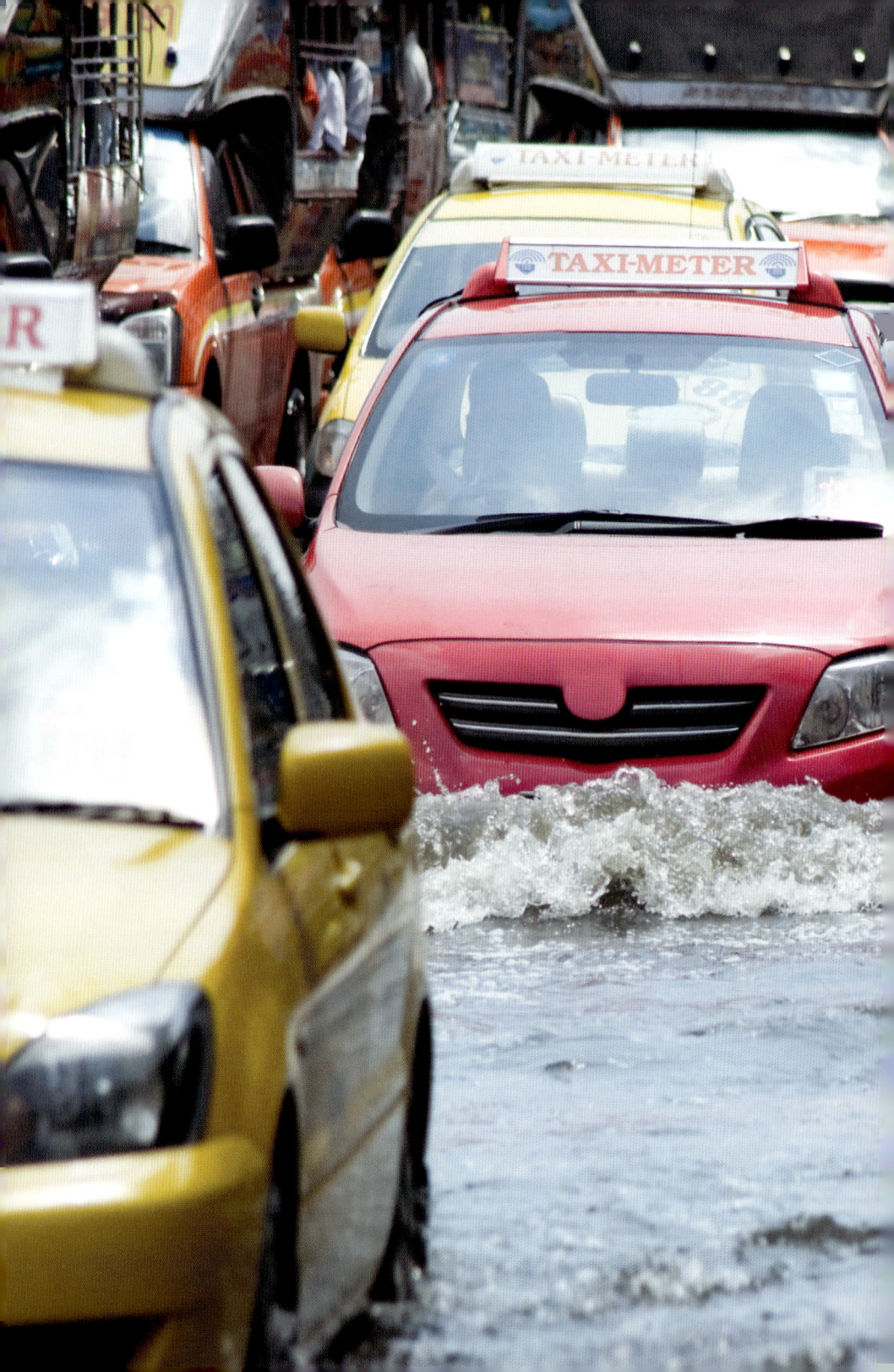

Keeping our heads above the water

Pawinee Kupatawintu, Thai National Stem Cell Donor Registry

In September 2011, there was a major flood in Bangkok; it was the first major flood the Thai National Stem Cell Donor Registry had to face since we were established in 2002.

Many organisations analysed flood information and we were no exception. Our problem was the liquid nitrogen tanks that stored our thousands of cord blood units, ready to be used for patients in need of a transplant. If the flood came, what would happen to this valuable inventory? With the help of modern technology, we were able to follow the situation as it developed and predict what would happen next. This helped us to make preparations, for example, by moving eight liquid nitrogen tanks containing cord blood units from the basement to a higher floor.

But during the flood and its aftermath, our first priority was the safety of our stem cell donors. After checking the list of appointments, we found that there were no urgent patient transplants in November 2011. So we consulted with the hospital and, with its approval, postponed all donor appointments to an unspecified later date.

By January 2012, the situation in Bangkok had returned to normal. We were able to start rescheduling appointments with our stem cell donors and could move the liquid nitrogen tanks back to the basement. Fortunately, they had suffered only minor damage.

While the flood was unfortunate, we know that experiences like these and the lessons we learned will help us to improve our ability to operate in the future.

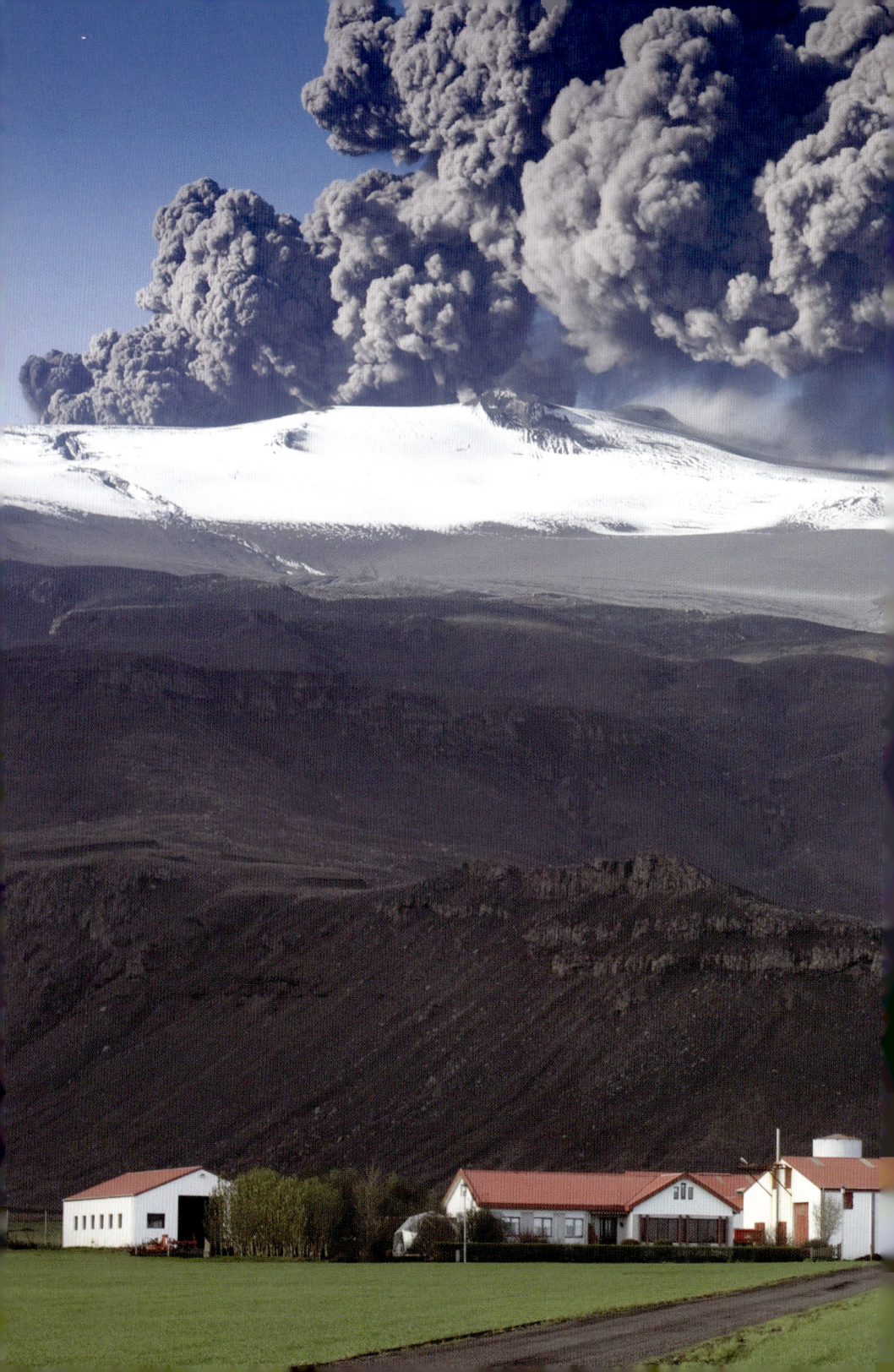

Collaboration across borders

Anne-Marie van Walraven, Search Consultant at Europdonor Foundation, the Netherlands

Do you remember Eyjafjallajökull? This Icelandic volcano erupted in April 2010, spewing huge amounts of ash into the atmosphere. Besides disrupting air travel for millions of holidaymakers and business travellers across Northern Europe, it also made work for us search coordinators much more complicated!

At Europdonor, we had scheduled a transportation of stem cells from Australia to the Netherlands for the week after the eruption. Our expectation was that the ash cloud would disappear over the weekend and that airspaces would reopen. In fact, we were so confident of this that we felt the recipient could begin with their pre-transplant conditioning treatment.

However, just one day later, it was announced that the European airspace would stay closed beyond the weekend. On that Sunday evening, my colleague Claire at the Australian Bone Marrow Donor Registry (ABMDR) called me at home to discuss the situation (it was already Monday for her). She had spoken to the donor and they were not able to donate the cells at a later date, but they did give their consent for the product to be cryopreserved.

Claire began to make the necessary arrangements at the collection centre and looked into how the cryopreserved product could be carried by hand. Neither of us had any experience with transporting cryopreserved cells, but we were certain that we would find a way. We expected airports to begin reopening on Tuesday. But Sally, another colleague from ABMDR, called just before midnight on

Monday to say the flight they had hoped to take had been cancelled. They were able to book a courier on to a flight on Wednesday. But that was subsequently also cancelled!

The courier was then booked on to a flight to New York, with the promise that they would be given first priority for the next flight to Madrid (which, by that point, was the closest accessible airport). The other option we investigated was transporting the cryopreserved product in a dry shipper with a professional courier company. But this turned out to be a no go too—shipment of liquid nitrogen in gas phase was purely for cargo and not medical products.

After countless phone calls back and forth to Australia, we realised we did not have much of a choice—we had to ship the product to Madrid. The final route would be from Brisbane to Sydney to Bangkok, and then to Madrid. The courier company agreed to send a car to pick up the product in Madrid and drive it 1,750 km back to the Netherlands.

Once these arrangements were in place, we were hoping we could relax a little. In our dreams! The next obstacle we encountered was that we needed an official permit to have the shipper cleared by Spanish customs. Sally called me on Tuesday night and said that the courier would not start the shipment without this permit.

> "Once these arrangements were in place, we were hoping we could relax a little. In our dreams!"

It was after 6pm in Europe and we were unable to reach our Spanish colleagues at the Spanish Redmo registry. I left a message on their answering machine, and asked Sally to speak to the courier and persuade them that a permit would be arranged upon arrival of the product in Spain. Sally made copies of all the paperwork, and I finally got through to Cecilia, our colleague in Spain, early the next morning. She kindly offered to take care of the permit for us (which included getting approval from the Ministry of Health).

Thanks to Cecilia's sharp organisational skills, we received the permit just two hours later. Airspace over the Netherlands was still closed, but with a car on its way to Spain, we could almost smell victory! We eventually received the shipment at noon on 23 April and, a few hours later, I hand-delivered the product to the hospital. The patient had the transplant two days later than planned, but fortunately, the procedure went smoothly.

For me, this story highlights how important the whole WMDA community is. If I ever have any problems or worries, I know I can turn to my colleagues in other countries—and for that I am very grateful.

> The WMDA has developed guidelines for establishing organisational resiliency programmes to deal with emergencies. These guidelines stress the need for international cooperation, as well as for prevention and mitigation, crisis response, business continuity and disaster recovery. They also require ongoing maintenance and revision.*
>
> *Extracted from Pingel et al, Biology of Blood and Marrow Transplantation (2012).

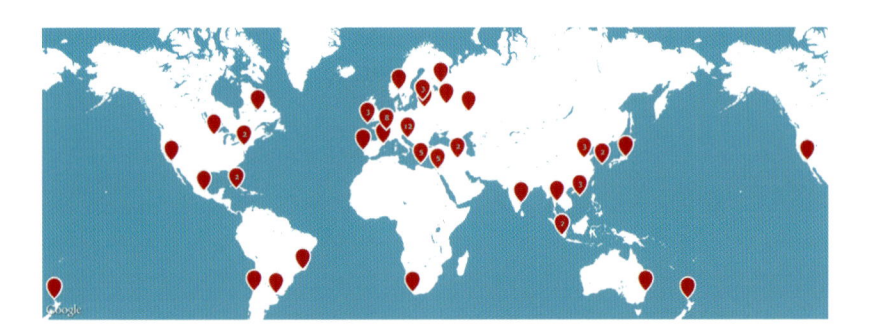

WMDA is celebrating a milestone: 25 million donors
Serving blood stem cell organisations worldwide

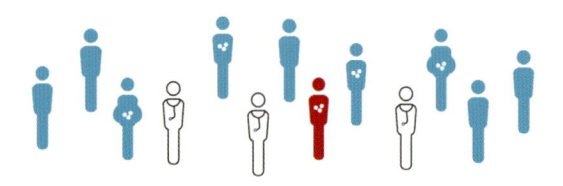

25,712,736
donors

1,145,000
transplantations

665,195
cord blood units

Corporate member:

MEMBERS	DONORS	PATIENTS	PROFESSIONALS	ABOUT US
SITEMAP	Who	Who	Starting a registry	Who we are
Disclaimer	Blood stem cells	Blood stem cells	Get involved	What we do
Map	Donation	Finding a donor	Accreditation	WMDA meetings
	Protection	Transplantation	Tools	Publications
	Risks	Risks	News	Join us
			Events and Calendar	Contact us

Summary

The stories in this book are a reality—they are happening every day.

What you have read is a wonderful example of how global cooperation has saved lives all over the world, through both the local and international exchange of stem cells. These efforts have had a genuine and lasting impact on the lives of patients and their families, as well as on their stem cell donors and the people who have been a part of facilitating that effort. We are always moved by how donors and stem cell couriers give their time, effort and a part of themselves in such a selfless manner.

We hope that you might choose to be a part of this worldwide effort. If you are eligible, sign up as a donor. If you are able to, take part in activities run by your local registry. Or if you can afford it, you can also help to fund your local registry or cord blood bank. Most of all, you can choose to live your life to the full while treasuring each and every moment—just as many of our patients have learned to.

Wherever you are and whatever you choose to do, we hope that this book has inspired you to seize, enjoy and share life in any way you can.

For more information, to become a donor or to find details of an unrelated blood cell donor registry or cord blood bank near you, please visit **www.wmda.info**.

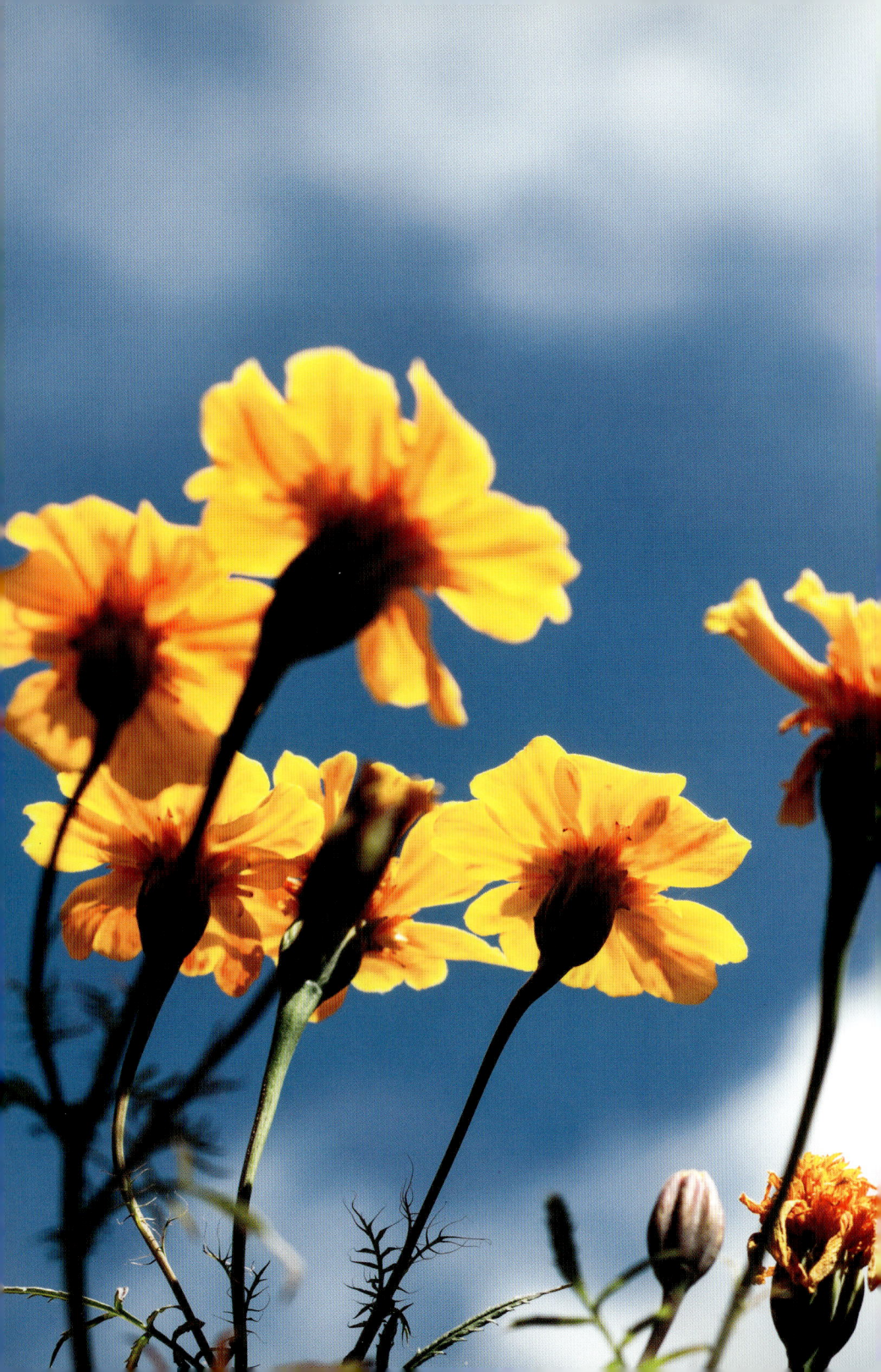

Acknowledgements

This book would not have been possible without the contributions of the following individuals and organisations who gave their time and effort to make it a reality.

- Our selfless authors, for their willingness to share a little bit about their lives.

- Lydia Foeken, Monique Jöris, Dorien de Kruijf and Daniela Orsini, the invaluable WMDA team members who contacted the authors of the stories, guided the project and brought it to fruition.

- Mei Hwang for her help in additional proofreading of the script.

- The translators Dr Linn Yeh Ching and Dr Ma Liyuan (Chinese); Mr Koh Chuan and Mdm Sato Yuriko (Japanese); and Ms Soon-ok Heijmans (Korean).

- The SingHealth Foundation and Singapore General Hospital, for their generous support in providing the initial funds that helped to kick-start the project.

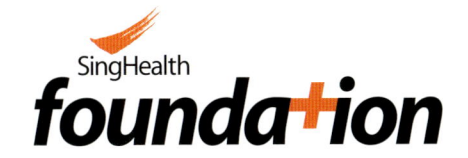

SingHealth founda+ion

Initial funds for this book was made possible by a generous grant from the SingHealth Foundation.

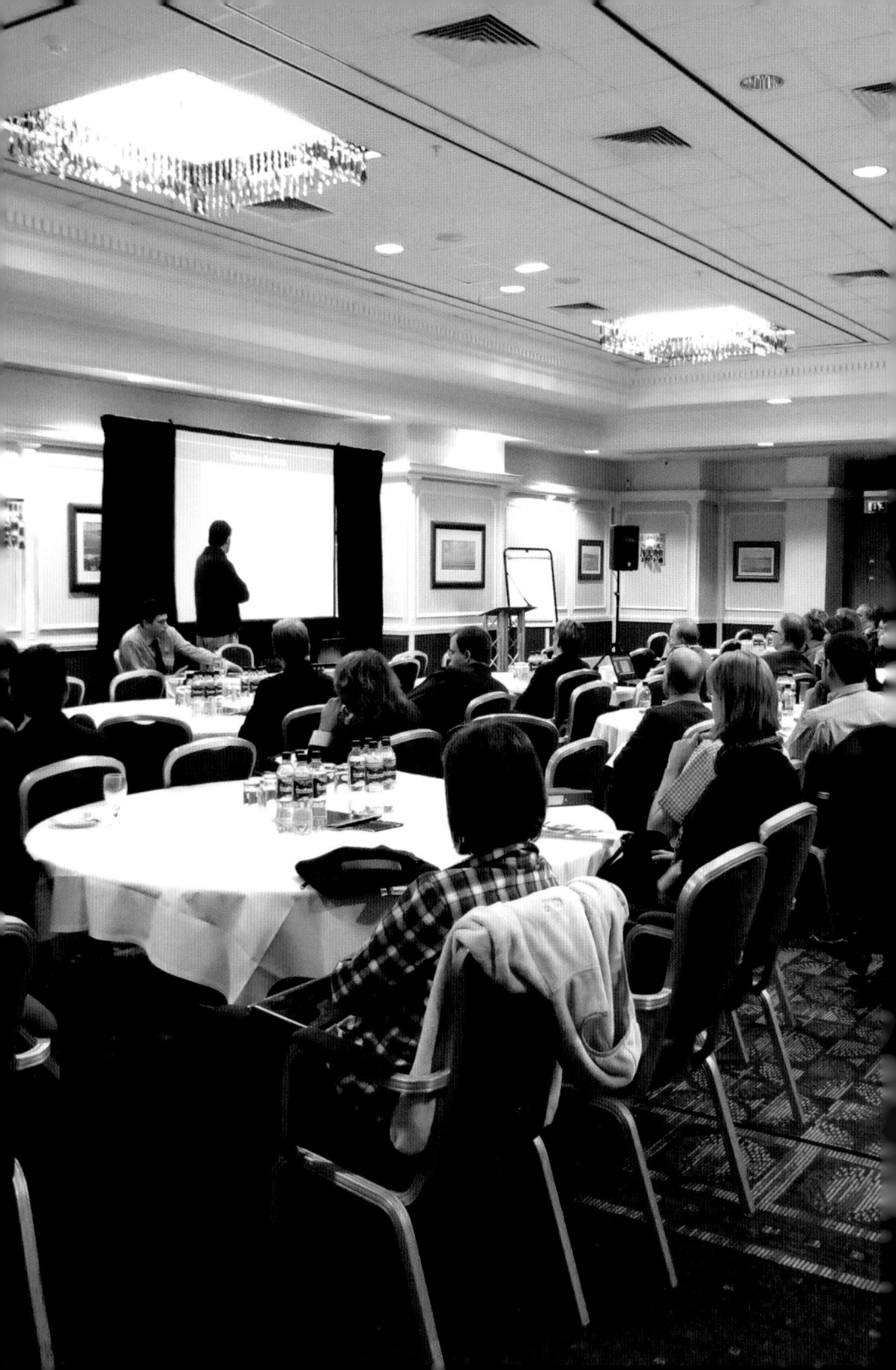

Contributing registries

Anthony Nolan
www.anthonynolan.org
Anthony Nolan is the UK's blood cancer charity and bone marrow register. It matches remarkable people willing to donate their stem cells to people in desperate need of a bone marrow or stem cell transplant. Since it was set up 40 years ago, the charity has given more than 13,000 people a new chance at life.

Armenian Bone Marrow Donor Registry
www.abmdr.am
The Armenian Bone Marrow Donor Registry (ABMDR) and its EFI-accredited HLA-typing laboratory was established in 1999. The ABMDR is a WMDA and BMDW participating donor registry and haematopoietic stem cell (HSC) collection centre. As a small country in the South Caucasus region, the ABMDR is a unique haematopoietic cells and bone marrow donor centre that uses genetic ancestry for better matches and outcomes.

Having been in the field for more than 14 years, it has been successful in mobilising, recruiting and creating a reliable donor database that now lists more than 26,000 potential donors not only from Armenia, but from people of Armenian descent worldwide. The registry is the only facility of its type among the former Soviet states. It has extensive experience of working closely with local communities and public organisations, and maintains close relationships with more than 65 HSC donor registries and a number of transplant centres in Europe and the US.

Australian Marrow Donors Registry
www.abmdr.org.au
The Australian Marrow Donors Registry (ABMDR) has grown from 6,000 donors in 1991 to 175,000 enrolled donors in 2014. Along with Gift of Life Australia, the ABMDR is responsible for recruiting volunteer bone marrow/blood stem cell donors in Australia. The ABMDR also has administrative management of the National Cord

Blood Collection Network (public cord blood banks). In 2013, 26 per cent of all donor collections were for international patients.

National Marrow Donor Program/Be The Match
www.bethematch.org
For people with life-threatening blood cancers like leukaemia and lymphoma, or other diseases, a cure exists. Be The Match connects patients with their donor match for a life-saving marrow or umbilical cord blood transplant. People can contribute to the cure as a member of the Be The Match Registry, financial contributor or volunteer. Be The Match provides patients and their families one-on-one support, education, and guidance before, during and after transplant. Be The Match is operated by the National Marrow Donor Program (NMDP), a non-profit organisation that matches patients with donors, educates health care professionals and conducts research so that more lives can be saved.

BIONET Corp
www.babybanks.com/2009/bionet-en/about_us.html
BIONET Corp was first established in 1999 as a pioneering company in the field of stem cell application in Taiwan and across Asia. BIONET has focused on stem cell therapy and genetic testing. In 2007, BIONET completed its initial public offering (TPO: 1784) and became the first publicly traded company in Taiwan's stem cell and genetics industry. Furthermore, in 2012, Genesis Genetics Asia Corp (GGA), a subsidiary of BIONET, made its IPO (TPO: 4160) as Taiwan's first public company specialising in both genetic testing and scientific informatics. BIONET Corp is Taiwan's largest enterprise for cell therapy and genetic engineering, with a penetration rate of up to nearly 50 per cent.

Bone Marrow Donor Programme Singapore
www.bmdp.org
The Bone Marrow Donor Programme (BMDP) is a non-profit organisation responsible for building and managing Singapore's only register of volunteer donors willing to give their bone marrow to save the lives of patients with leukaemia and other blood diseases. So far almost 500 patients have been given a chance of survival through the work of the BMDP, and the need grows every year as transplants become a routine treatment for these common forms of cancer.

Bone Marrow Registry in Nigeria
www.bonemarrownigeria.org
The Bone Marrow Registry in Nigeria (BMRN) is a non-profit organisation based at the University of Nigeria Teaching Hospital's College of Medicine in Enugu. It is the first internationally accredited donor registry in Nigeria, and only the second in Africa. Its mission is to improve access to genetically diverse stem cell donors from Nigeria, and to match them with patients all over the world. It is also seeking to construct the first cord blood bank in Africa in order to support haematopoietic stem cell research and transplantation.

Buddhist Tzu Chi Stem Cell Centre
http://btcscc.tzuchi.com.tw/btcscc_en
In 1992, Ms Wen Wen-ling, a student from Taiwan studying abroad in the US, developed leukaemia but was unable to find a match from banks in the US or Japan. Helpless, she decided to return to Taiwan to push for a change in legislation to allow for unrelated bone marrow transplants, hoping to find a chance for survival for both herself and other Chinese leukaemia patients overseas. In January 1993, despite her physical pain, she travelled to Hualien to visit Dharma Master Cheng Yen. During the meeting, she pleaded for Tzu Chi to help leukaemia patients by creating a registry of bone marrow donors in Taiwan.

In May of the same year, Legislative Yuan approved a revision of the Organ Transplant Statute which repealed the third-grade relative restriction on bone marrow donations. Following this, the Department of Health convened a special meeting on setting up a bone marrow donor database, and entrusted Tzu Chi with establishing and operating Taiwan's bone marrow donor registry. After Dharma Master Cheng Yen was given final assurance that saving lives through marrow transplantation presented no risk to a donor's health, Tzu Chi formally founded the registry in October 1993. Meanwhile, Tzu Chi volunteers across the country launched marrow donor sign-ups and donor blood testing drives.

In November 2005, Tzu Chi and Bone Marrow Donor Worldwide celebrated reaching the milestone of having 10 million donors in the international online donor registry. As of 2007, the centre had uploaded donor data for more than 300,000 people, which means that three out of every 100 donors in the database are from Taiwan.

In 2005, Tzu Chi Stem Cell Centre completed its 1,000th stem cell donation.

China Marrow Donor Program
www.cmdp.com.cn
Around 50,000 people are diagnosed with leukaemia every year in China. To respond to the growing demand for haematopoietic stem cell transplants, the Chinese government began funding the China Marrow Donor Program (CMDP) in 2001, and entrusted the Red Cross Society of China with its management. Like its American counterpart, the National Marrow Donor Program, CMDP works closely with the various systems already in place for donor recruitment, HLA typing, clinical transplant and the provision of stem cells to patients in other countries. CMDP currently has 31 regional branches, 30 HLA contract labs and 110 contract transplant centres across China. To date, 1,997,093 volunteer donors have registered with the CMDP. And it has helped 4,612 patients, including many outside China, to receive life-saving stem cells.

Czech National Marrow Donors Registry
www.kostnidren.cz/registry/index.html
The Czech National Marrow Donors Registry was established in 1992 as a non-governmental, non-profit organisation supported by the Bone Marrow Transplantation Foundation. In March 2005, it successfully achieved provisional accreditation by the WMDA. Full accreditation was granted after two on-site inspections in 2010 and 2014 (it remains the only WMDA-accredited registry among former Soviet states). The registry had 50,000 donors registered in September 2014, and as of 31 October 2014 it had facilitated 1,169 HSC donations, with 534 donations, for national and international patients.

Datri Blood Stem Cell Donors Registry
www.datriworld.org
Datri Blood Stem Cell Donors Registry was launched in India in 2009 by Raghu Rajagopal, Dr Nezih Cereb and Dr Soo Young Yang. Based in Chennai, Datri had more than 70,000 donors and had facilitated 78 donations in India as of November 2014. Its donors are spread across the country. Datri is registered with BMDW and is a member of the WMDA.

DKMS—German Bone Marrow Donor Centre
www.dkms.de/en
DKMS began with one family's search for a bone marrow donor. In 1990, Peter Harf and his daughters went from door to door to find a donor match for his wife and their mother, Mechtild Harf. They registered 68,000 donors in just one year. Sadly, Mechtild lost her battle, but in her honour the Harf family started a bone marrow donor centre that has since grown into the world's largest. DKMS has branches in the US, Germany, the UK, Poland and Spain. Globally, DKMS has registered more than 4.5 million donors and provided more than 40,000 patients with a second chance at life.

DONORMO—Mexican Bone Marrow Donors Registry
www.fundacioncompartevida.org.mx
DONORMO was created in 1998. It was the second registry established in Latin America and is the only one in Mexico. Its donors have been included in the BMDW database since 1999. DONORMO had 16,600 donors as of November 2014. However, for a country of 118 million people (according to 2011 census), this is insignificant; barely 1.4 donors per 10,000 people.

DONORMO has grown thanks to the hard work and commitment of its members and friends, and the patronage of The Fundación Comparte Vida. It has facilitated 125 bone marrow transplants using unrelated units (for national and international patients, receiving and shipping products) and supports more than 60 per cent of the HLA donor-recipient selection for family members performed in Mexico.

Ezer Mizion
www.ezermizion.org
Ezer Mizion is one of Israel's largest and most highly respected non-profit health support organisations. It offers a broad scope of programmes that serve every segment of Israel's population. Ezer Mizion's flagship project is its bone marrow registry, which is the world's fifth largest, and provides extensive support services to cancer patients and their families.

Europdonor
www.europdonor.nl/
Europdonor helps doctors find a suitable donor of life-saving stem cells extracted from bone marrow. To ensure the successful treatment of life-threatening blood diseases, it maintains a record of Dutch stem cell donors, cooperates with international partners and performs its own scientific research. It also offers both medical professionals and the public education and information. Together with the Sanquin Blood Supply Foundation, it actively recruits new donors in the fight against a number of life-threatening diseases. A non-profit organisation, Europdonor was founded in 1988 by the passionate physician and researcher Prof Dr Jon van Rood. As one of the early pioneers in the field of transplantation in the Netherlands, he was among the first to identify the opportunities for unrelated stem cell transplantation. To this day, Europdonor continues to benefit from his counsel and support.

Finnish Stem Cell Registry
http://www.veripalvelu.fi/www/StemCellRegistry
The Finnish Stem Cell Registry is a part of the Finnish Red Cross Blood Service and has been operating since 1992. It currently contains the details of some 25,000 potential donors. Around 500 Finnish registry members have donated their bone marrow or blood stem cells to date. The registry's services are available to all hospitals in Finland and abroad.

Gift of Life Bone Marrow Foundation
www.giftoflife.org
The Gift of Life Bone Marrow Foundation is a public donor registry based in the US that serves patients worldwide in need of transplants. Gift of Life is accredited by the WMDA. At the time of writing, it had 234,429 registered donors and had undertaken 69,822 patient searches, with matches being found for 11,471 patients. As a result of this, 2,791 transplants have been facilitated, giving many people the gift of a second chance at life.

Hadassah Medical Centre
www.hadassahinternational.org
The Arab Donor Project is a programme operated by Hadassah Medical Centre Bone Marrow and Cord Blood Donor Registry, which

was established by Prof Chaim Brautbar in 1987. Today the registry has more than 125,500 potential donors and 9,236 cord blood units, and is headed by Dr Shoshanna Israel.

The Arab Donor Project was launched in 2008 by Dr Amal Bishara and Prof Chaim Brautbar in order to recruit Arab donors to the Hadassah registry. All recruitment activities and public relations among the 1.7 million Arabs in Israel are managed by Dr Amal Bishara.

The number of Arab donors listed in the registry increased from 130 in 2008 to more than 30,000 in 2014. Hundreds of these have been matched with Arab and non-Arab donors locally and worldwide, with 44 donors going on to donate bone marrow/stem cells.

Japan Marrow Donor Program
www.jmdp.or.jp/english.html
The Japan Marrow Donor Program (JMDP) was established in 1991 as a cooperation with the Japanese Red Cross Society under a government initiative. Since the first unrelated bone marrow transplant in 1993, more than 14,800 transplants have been performed. As of October 2012, the number of registered donors exceeded 419,000, and these donors have A/B/DR serological or DNA data. JMDP is a participating registry in BMDW and is certified by the WMDA. It cooperates with a huge number of foreign registries to save patients with blood diseases around the world.

Korean Marrow Donor Program
http://www.kmdp.or.kr
The Korean Marrow Donor Program (KMDP) was established in March 1994 and, as of June 2014, had 273,785 stem cell donors listed. KMDP has provided stem cells to more than 3,400 patients in need.

New Zealand Bone Marrow Donor Registry
www.bonemarrow.org.nz
The New Zealand Bone Marrow Donor Registry (NZBMDR) is managed by the Leukaemia & Blood Foundation and works very closely with the New Zealand Blood Service and tissue typing laboratory, as well as transplant centres nationwide. It has

approximately 1,2000 potential donors who are willing to donate cells from their bone marrow to patients worldwide, if they are ever found to be a match.

South African Bone Marrow Registry
www.sabmr.co.za
The South African Bone Marrow Registry (SABMR) was created by Prof Ernette du Toit and Prof Peter Jacobs in 1991. In the same year, it was approved as a member of the WMDA and designated an internationally recognised registry.

The SABMR is the only bone marrow registry in South Africa. It has more than 65,000 South African donors in its database and access to more than 20 million donors worldwide through its international association with the WMDA. Since it launched, the SABMR has conducted searches to identify donors for more than 1,500 children and adults.

Stefan Morsch Foundation
http://en.stefan-morsch-stiftung.com/index.php
The Stefan Morsch Foundation currently has around 408,000 donors registered in Germany and a further 6,000 registered in Luxembourg. When the foundation started to increase the number of donors in its database, the need arose for an HLA laboratory that could handle the huge volume of blood samples. This led to the establishment of its EFI and ASHI-accredited laboratory in 1997.

Since January 2003, the foundation's International Donor Search Centre has been searching worldwide for matched donors for patients in Russia and Jordan, and in 2013 it expanded its activities for German transplant centres. To date, the Stefan Morsch Foundation has been able to identify more than 1,000 matching donors from around the world. In 2005 it opened its own adult stem cell collection centre in Birkenfeld, Germany, to collect peripheral stem cells and donor lymphocytes for use in allogeneic transplants.

Swiss Transfusion SRC (Swiss Red Cross)
http://en.blutspende.ch/index.php
In 1988, the Swiss bone marrow donor registry was established by a group of private individuals from the spheres of blood stem cell transplantation, blood transfusion and medicine. That same year,

the first bone marrow transplant using cells from a foreign donor was performed. The central functions of Swiss Blood Stem Cells, a part of Swiss Transfusion SRC, are managing the registry of blood stem cell donors in Switzerland, recruiting donors in Switzerland, and coordinating donations by donors in Switzerland for patients in Switzerland and abroad. Blood stem cell transplantation is often the only hope of a cure for people suffering from a malignant blood disease like leukaemia.

Thai National Stem Cell Donor Registry
www.stemcellthairedcross.com
The Thai National Stem Cell Donor Registry was established in 2002. It was launched after one Thai patient could not find a donor among their relatives, and tried to recruit an unrelated donor from their group of friends and wider society. The Thai Red Cross became aware of the situation and a need to help similar patients. The Thai National Stem Cell Donor Registry is the only official registry in Thailand.

LA
LLAM

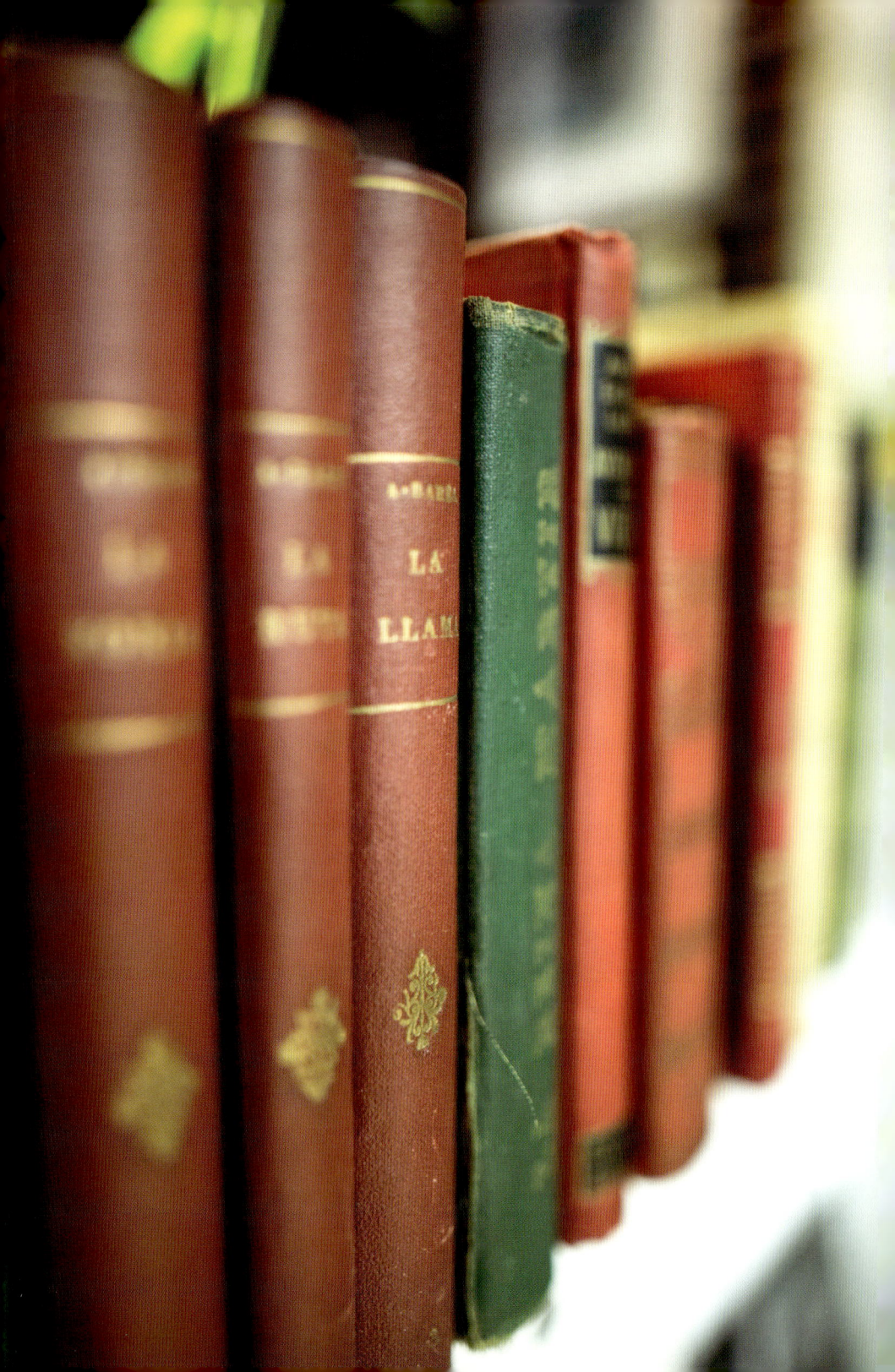

Glossary

Allogeneic
A term usually used in organ or stem cell transplants. It means 'from another person'. An allogeneic transplant is, therefore, a transplant using an organ or cells from another person.

Apheresis/pheresis
The process by which blood is collected and run through a machine which separates the blood into various components via centrifugation. The desired blood component is then extracted while the rest of the blood is returned to the patient in real time. Depending on how the machine is configured, donors can donate either platelets or white blood cells. For peripheral blood stem cell donation, the white blood cell fraction is extracted while the rest of the blood is returned.

ASHI
The American Society for Histocompatibility and Immunogenetics is an international society of professionals dedicated to advancing the science, education and application of immunogenetics and transplant immunology.

Autologous
Also a term usually used in organ or stem cell transplants. It means 'from self'. An autologous transplant is, therefore, a transplant using an organ or cells from one's own body.

Blood bank*
Medical facility where blood intended for transfusion is drawn and stored.

Blood stem cell transplant
(Sometimes called 'haematopoietic stem cell transplant', but not to be confused with peripheral blood stem cell transplant, which is a subset of this)

The process where a patient undergoes some form of preparative therapy comprising of chemotherapy with/without radiotherapy to reduce the number of tumour and immune cells, followed by infusion of donor cells to the patient. If the donor cells are obtained from the bone marrow, this is sometimes called a bone marrow transplant (BMT); if collected from the blood, it is sometimes called a peripheral blood stem cell transplant (PBSCT). And if donor cells come from umbilical cord blood, this is often referred to as a cord blood transplant (CBT).

Bone marrow
The inner spongy tissue present within bones (especially around the pelvis and sternum) which serves as a 'factory' that produces all the essential blood cells, including white blood cells (which help fight infection), red blood cells (which help carry oxygen) and platelets (which help stop bleeding). Bone marrow can be extracted in small amounts for diagnostic purposes (to determine if any bone marrow related blood disorder exists) or in larger quantities as part of a standard bone marrow harvest for donation to another individual. Bone marrow cells usually self-replenish very quickly.

BMDW
Stands for bone marrow donors worldwide. BMDW is a voluntary collaborative effort of stem cell donor registries and cord blood banks whose goal is to provide centralised information on the HLA phenotypes and other relevant data of unrelated stem cell donors and cord blood units and to make this information easily accessible to the physicians of patients in need of a hematopoietic stem cell transplant.

Bone marrow transplant
See 'Blood stem cell transplant'.

Central venous catheter/line
Venous catheters that are placed, by trained personnel, into central veins below the clavicle or neck to help facilitate the infusion of drugs and the collection of blood for various tests. The insertion of these lines is usually under the assistance of some radiological imaging. Larger catheters, called apheresis lines, may be used for

collecting large volumes of blood for stem cell harvesting (these are not unlike the dialysis catheters used for dialysis or patients with kidney failure).

Collection centre*
Medical facility where haematopoietic stem cell collection from selected donors takes place. This collection process might include marrow aspiration or apheresis. The collection centre performs the medical workup of the donor and provides final approval of the donor for harvest. If umbilical cord blood is collected, the centre is responsible for processing and storing the cord blood unit. In the context of cord blood banks, this usually refers to the obstetric hospital where the cord blood is collected.

Cord blood/umbilical cord blood
Blood taken from the umbilical cord of a baby after the child is delivered and the cord has been clamped and cut. Therefore, collection takes place after the umbilical cord is separated and should have no effect on the baby. Usually, the blood is collected by needle or another device that draws blood from the umbilical cord and placenta into a blood bag or other form of sterile container (after the baby has been taken aside to be looked after by delivery room staff). These cells have been found to be rich in blood stem cells and therefore a useful source of cells for transplantation. Unlike bone marrow transplants, cord blood transplants are associated with the slower recovery of blood counts (due to the smaller numbers of cells) but with a lower incidence of graft-versus-host disease (see below).

Cord blood bank*
A donor centre whose sole purpose is to collect and maintain umbilical cord blood units, and which may combine some or all of the activities of both a donor centre and a collection centre. For example, a cord blood bank may be responsible for donor recruitment, cord blood collection and storage, but the database of donors might be maintained by a registry. Alternatively, the cord blood bank might perform all of these activities and carry out searches for transplant centres.

Courier
In the context of this book, couriers are individuals who accompany blood stem cell products from a collection centre to a transplant centre. Many couriers are volunteers, though some professional couriers may also be used. For cord blood shipments involving the use of a liquid nitrogen shipper, professional couriers are usually contracted.

Donors*
Donors are defined as (1) volunteer adult donors of haematopoietic stem cells or (2) umbilical cord blood units collected after maternal permission.

Donor centre*
An institution responsible for recruiting, gaining the consent of, counselling, and coordinating the testing of potential donors. It monitors the short and long-term health of adult volunteer donors who have provided haematopoietic stem cells. It also maintains a register or database of donors, which may be searched as appropriate.

EFI
The European federation for immunogenetics promotes education and information exchange between professionals working in immunogenetics research field.

G-CSF
Stands for granulocyte-colony stimulating factor. This is used to stimulate the bone marrow to produce stem cells and release them into the donor's bloodstream before collection by leukapheresis.

Genotype
The genetic make-up of an organism or group of organisms with reference to a single trait, set of traits or an entire complex of traits. In this book we talk about the genetic make-up of the immune system.

Graft-versus-host disease (GVHD)
Condition where a donor's immune cells attack the patient. This can happen even in a fully matched HLA transplant, as there are many other minor tissue differences possible between two individuals

who are not identical twins. GVHD can occur acutely (usually early post-transplant) or chronically (usually occurring later on). Acute GVHD usually manifests with diarrhoea, liver dysfunction and a skin rash. Chronic GVHD may manifest in a variety of ways, including dry eyes, a dry mouth, as well as stiff skin and joints. There are good treatments options available for GVHD.

Haematopoietic
'Haema' means blood. 'Haematopoietic' therefore means 'blood forming'. For simplicity, the terms haematopoietic stem cell and blood stem cell are used interchangeably in this book. Peripheral blood stem cells, however, refer exclusively to blood stem cells harvested from the peripheral blood.

Haematopoietic stem cell
Blood-derived stem cells are cells which are capable of surviving for a very long time while producing daughter cells of many different types, as well as reproducing exact copies of themselves. In adults, the majority of these cells reside in the bone marrow unless they are stimulated. In this case, the daughter cells that they produce are red blood cells, platelets and the various white blood cells.

Haematopoietic stem cell transplant
For the purposes of this book, which is catered to a wide readership, this term is used synonymously with the term 'blood stem cell transplant'.

Harvest (bone marrow or peripheral blood stem cells)
The process by which cells are collected from the donor. Bone marrow harvests are usually performed in the operating theatre, where bone marrow is collected from pelvic bones under general anaesthesia. Peripheral blood stem cell harvests are conducted using an apheresis machine, which collects the white blood cells while returning the rest of the blood to the donor. Collection of these stem cells is made possible by the prior injection of drugs such as G-CSF.

Human leukocyte antigen (HLA)
Cell proteins found on the surface of white blood cells which help to determine tissue compatibility when transplants are performed. These proteins are important in determining the compatibility of

tissues because white blood cells are inherently immune cells which function in rejecting cells that appear foreign to the body. Therefore, a HLA match minimises the chances that the immune cells of patient and donor reject one another.

Matched sibling
A sibling of a patient who is fully matched to the patient in all the desired HLA loci. If the sibling is found fit and willing to donate, then the sibling becomes a matched sibling donor.

Matched unrelated donor
A stem cell donor who is not a close relative of the patient, but who is fully matched to the patient in all the desired HLA loci. A full match ensures the best compatibility in the cells of the two individuals.

Mismatched donor
A donor of stem cells who is not fully matched to the patient in all the desired HLA loci. A mismatch increases the risk of complications because the immune cells of the donor have a greater chance of attacking the patient and vice versa.

Neutrophils
A type of white blood cell that forms an essential part of the immune system. They are normally found in the bloodstream and are one of the first cell types to travel to the site of infection.

Peripheral blood
Blood that may be obtained from the peripheral veins of the body.

Peripheral blood stem cell
Haematopoietic stem and progenitor cells that may be obtained from the peripheral veins. These cells are usually coaxed out of the bone marrow by injecting drugs such as G-CSF. This is a drug with a long safety record and which has also been used to help accelerate the recovery of white blood cells in patients who have received chemotherapy.

Peripheral blood stem cell transplant
See 'Blood stem cell transplant'.

Platelets
Cell fragments which go to sites of bleeding within the body in order to stop the blood loss by plugging the gap and initiating blood clotting.

Recruitment centre
Centre where donors are recruited for enrolment into a bone marrow/blood stem cell registry.

Red blood cells
Blood cells which help carry oxygen around the body. These cells give blood its red colour, which comes from the high levels of haemoglobin and iron within these cells.

Registry*
A Registry is a national organisation whose responsibility it is to process requests for haematopoietic stem cells from donors originating from within the country and from abroad. A registry may coordinate the activities of donor, collection and transplant centres in its respective country.

Shipper
In this book this term is used to refer to containers used to hold blood stem cell products during transportation of cells between two centres. Insulated cooler boxes, not unlike those used to transport blood, are commonly used. Sometimes, cold packs (unfrozen and without direct contact with the blood bag) may be used to help maintain a consistent temperature. If the stem cells are already frozen, as is usually the case with cord blood when it is shipped from cord blood banks to transplant centres, miniature liquid nitrogen tanks with temperature monitoring and approved to withstand such shipments will be used.

Stem cells
Cells which are capable of surviving for a very long time while producing daughter cells of many different types as well as reproducing exact copies of themselves.

Testing laboratory*
These laboratories perform the histocompatibility, blood group, infectious diseases and other testing for potential donors and patients. They may be under the direction of a registry, donor centre or transplant centre, or may be separate from these entities.

Transplant centre*
The medical facility where a patient (recipient) receives a transplant (graft) with haematopoietic stem cells from an unrelated donor or from an umbilical cord blood unit. The centre oversees the immediate medical treatment and provides long-term follow-up of the recipient. A 'search unit' undertakes searches for unrelated donors for specific patients. This entity may be contained within a transplant centre, or may be separate from the centre. If separate, the search unit may coordinate searches for one or several transplant centres. Transplant centres/search units seeking international donors work through the registry in their country.

Verification typing*
The tests carried out on a specific donor at the request of a transplant centre to determine the appropriateness of using haematopoietic stem cells from that donor for a specific patient.

White blood cells
Blood cells which help us to fight infection. These comprise neutrophils (which form a first line of blood immunity), lymphocytes (which are capable of more specific responses) and many other cells. Blood stem cells are white blood cells and are often found in this blood compartment.

Workup*
At this stage, a volunteer has been identified as a match for a patient, agrees to donate haematopoietic stem cells, and is medically evaluated for his or her fitness to donate stem cells.

Definition extracted and adapted from Hurley et al, Bone Marrow Transplantation (2004) 34, 103–110.

Notes

Notes